Clinical Thermology

Subseries Thermotherapy

M. Gautherie (Ed.)

Interstitial, Endocavitary and Perfusional Hyperthermia

Methods and Clinical Trials

With Contributions by
J.M. Cosset · K.-H. Bichler · W.L. Strohmaier · J. Steimann
S.H. Flüchter · K. Sugimachi · H. Matsuda · F. Truchetet
E. Grosshans · J.C. Kretz · J. Friedel · C. Chartier

With 55 Figures and 33 Tables

Springer-Verlag Berlin Heidelberg New York
London Paris Tokyo Hong Kong

Dr. Michel Gautherie
Laboratoire de Thermologie Biomédicale
Université Louis Pasteur
Institut National de la Santé
et de la Recherche Médicale
11, rue Humann
67085 Strasbourg Cedex, France

Library of Congress Cataloging-in-Publication Data
Interstitial, endocavitary, and perfusional hyperthermia: methods and clinical trials / M. Gautherie, ed.; with contributions by J.M. Cosset ... [et al.]. p. cm. – (Clinical thermology. Subseries thermotherapy) Includes bibliographical references.
ISBN-13: 978-3-642-74642-0 e-ISBN-13: 978-3-642-74640-6
DOI: 10.1007/978-3-642-74640-6
1. Cancer – Thermotherapy. I. Gautherie, Michel. II. Cosset, J. M. III. Series.
RC271.T5I578 1990 616.99'40632 – dc 20 89-21969

Softcover reprint of the hardcover 1st edition 1990

Typesetting: K+V Fotosatz GmbH, Beerfelden

2127/3145-543210 – Printed on acid-free paper

Preface

"Internal" hyperthermia is a type of thermotherapy by which heat is supplied to tumor tissue in situ. There are three different techniques for providing internal hyperthermia: (1) interstitial hyperthermia using implanted needle probes, (2) intracavitary hyperthermia using probes introduced into natural body cavities, and (3) perfusional hyperthermia by means of extracorporal blood heating. Compared with external hyperthermia, internal hyperthermia has been preferentially accepted by oncologists because it can be more easily combined with other forms of treatment, e.g., interstitial thermotherapy with brachytherapy, or perfusional hyperthermia with chemotherapy.

Various types of equipment for interstitial and intracavitary thermotherapy have been developed and used quite extensively in clinical trials, generally in combination with radiation therapy. There are four different methods for producing interstitial or intracavitary hyperthermia, each related to different types of heating. Most studies have been performed using radiofrequency electrodes (resistive heating) or coaxial microwave antennas (radiative heating). Recently, however, "hot source" techniques that rely on thermal conduction and blood flow convection for heat transport have found clinical application. These techniques include ferromagnetic implants activated by hot water or by electrical means. In the near future, new methods for interstitial or intraluminal heating based upon advanced ultrasonic and laser technologies will be developed.

The principal advantage of interstitial and intracavitary thermotherapy is that, in contrast to external hyperthermia, power deposition can be restricted to the tumor site. This minimizes toxicities of various kinds that result from unwanted power deposition in normal tissues surrounding the tumor. Moreover, additional probe implantation for thermal dosimetry can be avoided by, for example, (a) inserting thermometric probes in hollow needle electrodes or water tubes, (b) using the same microwave antennas for radiometric temperature measurements, or (c) using self-thermoregulating seeds made of ferromagnetic materials whose Curie point is close to the required tumor temperature.

Despite the need for special interstitial probes and intraluminal applicators specifically designed for tumors in different anatomic locations, existing equipment permits performance of phase I and II clinical trials under good conditions. The present volume presents the technical and clinical state of the art in interstitial hyperthermia, and gives examples of applications of the other methods of internal hyperthermia in areas of major clinical interest in oncology, i.e., intracavitary hyperthermia in the treatment of cancers of the prostate, bladder, and esophagus, and perfusional hyperthermia in the treatment of malignant melanomas.

Strasbourg, Januar 1990 M. Gautherie

Contents

List of Contributors

K.-H. BICHLER
Universität Tübingen, Lehrstuhl und Abteilung für Urologie, Calwer Str. 7, 7400 Tübingen, West Germany

C. CHARTIER
Clinique Dermatologique, Hospices Civils, 67000 Strasbourg, France

J.M. COSSET
Institut Gustave Roussy, Rue Camille Desmoulins, 94805 Villejuif Cedex, France

S.H. FLÜCHTER
Universität Tübingen, Abteilung für Urologie, Calwer Str. 7, 7400 Tübingen, West Germany

J. FRIEDEL
Clinique Dermatologique, Hospices Civils, 67000 Strasbourg, France

E. GROSSHANS
Clinique Dermatologique, Hospices Civils, 67000 Strasbourg, France

J.C. KRETZ
Clinique Dermatologique, Hospices Civils, 67000 Strasbourg, France

H. MATSUDA
Department of Surgery II, Faculty of Medicine, Kyushu University, Fukuoka 812, Japan

J. STEIMANN
Universität Tübingen, Abteilung für Urologie, Calwer Str. 7, 7400 Tübingen, West Germany

W.L. STROHMAIER
Universität Tübingen, Abteilung für Urologie, Calwer Str. 7, 7400 Tübingen, West Germany

K. SUGIMACHI
Department of Surgery II, Faculty of Medicine, Kyushu University, Fukuoka 812, Japan

F. TRUCHETET
Service de Dermatologie, Hôpital Beauregard, rue des Frères, 57100 Thionville, France

1 Interstitial Hyperthermia

J.M. COSSET

1.1 Introduction

We can read in a document which was written 5000 years ago, and which is now known as the *Edwin Smith Surgical Papyrus*, the following sentence: "One having tumors in his breast... which I will treat with the fire drill..." [20, 96]. This is perhaps the first report concerning an attempt to treat a cancer using some kind of interstitial hyperthermia.

Since that time, different types of implantation or application of diverse hot materials have been attempted throughout the centuries in the hope of curing malignant tumors. However, in most cases these attempts should be regarded as cautery, and cannot really be equated with present-day interstitial heating [27].

In fact, interstitial hyperthermia really began in 1975, at the first International Symposium on Cancer Therapy by Hyperthermia and Radiation, when J. Doss [45, 46] proposed heating tumors between two arrays of implanted needles connected to a low frequency amplifier. At that time, most of the groups dealing with hyperthermia clearly preferred to utilize "external" techniques to treat their patients. For the radiation oncologists, essentially for those who were not used to brachytherapy, it appeared simpler to use a machine located "outside" the patient than to implant some type of invasive heating material.

Thus, only a few groups throughout the world took up the challenge of interstitial hyperthermia. The group at Tucson (University of Arizona) first demonstrated that, as for the other techniques of hyperthermia [14], interstitial heating used alone could not usually achieve the long-term control of a tumor, even when a complete regression was initially obtained [82]. This was confirmed shortly afterwards by the French group from Villejuif [29]. Consequently, a combination of interstitial hyperthermia and irradiation was very soon considered. Although external irradiation has sometimes been employed in conjunction with interstitial heating, most groups have developed combinations of interstitial hyperthermia and brachytherapy. There are at least three reasons for this; (a) it has seemed logical to combine these two invasive techniques, the only problem being to design a compatible system; (b) brachytherapy, with its continuous low dose rate irradiation, is known to be able to deliver tumoricidal doses with good normal tissue tolerance, and (c) some experimental data have suggested that the combination of hyperthermia and low dose rate irradiation was not only quite effective in controlling the tumor but also well tolerated by the surrounding normal tissues in laboratory animals [9, 10, 67, 90, 116]. However, a subsequent report by Gerner in 1983 [61] failed to confirm the importance of the irradiation dose rate over the range of standard interstitial radiation or external beam radiation therapy.

The preliminary technical and clinical data reported by the Tucson group were promising [82]. In parallel, other groups started to take an interest in interstitial hyperthermia for a variety of reasons. Some were impressed by the early Tucson results. Others were becoming somewhat disillusioned by the frequent failure of the external methods to deliver reliably an adequate thermal dose to the tumor volume in the anatomical sites concerned. In France, the long historical tradition of brachytherapy made it inevitable that there would be a strong interest in interstitial hyperthermia. Thus several teams began so use interstitial low frequency resistive diathermy, as proposed by Doss and developed in Tucson, either in the same way [53, 54, 55, 72, 77, 136, 138, 139, 143] or with slightly modified techniques [22, 31, 32, 34, 40, 58, 78].

Other centers preferred to develop a different procedure for interstitial thermotherapy, using *radiative* heating by means of microwave antennae, the frequency being in the range 300–1000 MHz. This technique was also usually combined with brachytherapy [2, 12, 13, 38–41, 53, 54, 55, 62, 93, 100, 106, 111, 124, 126, 127, 131, 134, 135, 142].

In addition, two groups in the United States have recently started to study implanted ferromagnetic seeds that can be inductively heated by a high frequency magnetic field [7, 21, 42, 80, 120]. So far this technique has not been applied to patients, but interesting results have been obtained for spontaneous tumors in pet animals [59].

From the data obtained in all those various centers, it was seen that interstitial techniques were capable of achieving the required tumor temperature increase (up to 42 °–44 °C) in a large number of cases. In addition, the distribution of temperature was usually satisfactory, with acceptable temperature inhomogeneities from point to point in the heated volume [28, 30, 52].

These technological advances, combined with the interesting preliminary clinical results, probably explain the present increasing interest in interstitial thermoradiotherapy. At the international hyperthermia meeting held in Fort Collins (U.S.A.) in 1980, only a few papers dealt with invasive techniques and the clinical results were scarce. Four years later, at the international meeting at Aarhus (Denmark), twenty posters and communications concerning interstitial hyperthermia were presented [95].

In his summary lecture on the clinical studies presented at this same symposium, N. Bleehen [14] wrote: "Interstitial thermoradiotherapy ... does currently seem to be the only technique for providing reasonably uniform heating in a smallish volume which is not actually at or very close to the surface ...".

In this chapter we will first consider the physical and technological aspects of interstitial hyperthermia. Then a detailed study of the available clinical results will lead us to the future prospects for this promising technique.

1.2 Physical and Technological Aspects of Interstitial Hyperthermia

Since the basic physical concepts of hyperthermia have already been extensively studied in a previous book of this series, we shall concentrate here on the specific features of interstitial heating, and particularly on the parameters directly related to the clinical applications.

As the physical principles and technological aspects are so closely linked, they are dealt with together in integrated sections as follows:

1. Resistive radiofrequency (low frequency) interstitial heating
2. Radiative microwave interstitial heating
3. Inductively heated ferromagnetic seeds
4. Other techniques

For this section, we shall essentially rely on the works of J. Strohbehn [121–123], T. Cetas [24, 25, 98], G. Hahn [65, 66], G. Nussbaum [91–93], L. Anghileri and J. Robert [1] and on the studies which were performed at the Institut Gustave-Roussy of Villejuif by J. Dutreix [49, 50].

1.2.1 Resistive Radiofrequency (Low Frequency) Interstitial Heating (RF Technique)

1.2.1.1 Physical Aspects

It is quite easy to induce a current between two electrodes implanted in (or located on both sides of) living tissue. If the frequency is low, more precisely if $w \cdot \varepsilon \ll \sigma$ (where w = angular frequency, ε = permittivity, and σ = electrical conductivity), the tissues behave in a purely resistive way. That is to say that the only currents flowing in those tissues are in phase with the applied voltage, the displacement currents being negligible. These conditions are met in soft tissues up to 100 MHz. It is worth noting that heating at RF is predominantly achieved by extracellular ions, while at low microwave frequencies heating is achieved by both extra- and intracellular ions. The various groups working throughout the world with frequencies in the range of 0.5–1 MHz are thus dealing with purely resistive heating.

Several parameters govern the distribution of the temperature throughout a volume heated by means of a resistive interstitial technique. One of the most important is obviously the *distribution of the power deposition*, expressed either per unit volume [absorption rate density (ARD) in $W\,m^{-3}$] or per unit mass [specific absorption rate (SAR) in $W\,kg^{-1}$]. The ARD and SAR are similar for most tissues , where density is near $1\ g\,cm^{-3}$, but they are different for some tissues of lower density, such as the lung.

The magnitude and spatial variation of this parameter are influenced by:

1. The voltage applied to the implanted electrodes
2. The electrical conductivity of the implanted tissues
3. The shape and size of the electrodes

In particular, conductivity varies widely from one tissue to another and may markedly affect the distribution of the SAR.

The conductivity of different tissue samples has been measured at 1 MHz by Hahn et al. [66] and Cosset et al. [29]. Similar results have been obtained by these two authors for blood: Hahn found σ (blood) = 7.6×10^{-3} mho-cm^{-1} (or $0.76\ S\,m^{-1}$), while Cosset reported σ (blood) = 6.45×10^{-3} mho-cm^{-1} (or

$0.64\,\mathrm{S\,m^{-1}}$). The results remain in acceptable agreement for muscle: Hahn reported σ (muscle) $= 5.8\times10^{-3}$ mho-cm^{-1}, while Cosset reported σ (muscle) $= 8.47\times10^{-3}$ mho-cm^{-1}. However, when considering fatty tissues, a discrepancy is observed: Hahn published σ (fat) $= 1.6\times10^{-3}$ mho-cm^{-1} (in fact with a wide range), whereas Cosset found a lower value: σ (fat) $= 0.23\times10^{-3}$ mho-cm^{-1}. This discrepancy could be explained by the fact that Hahn was working on human fatty tissues whereas Cosset studied pig fatty samples. On the other hand, while Hahn measured the conductivity on living tissues, Cosset used postmortem pig tissues, and we would have expected a higher conductivity in the latter case, because of the breakdown of (insulating) cell membranes. However, the presence of vascularization (see above the values of σ for blood, obviously higher than those for fatty tissues) could possibly account for a higher conductivity in the living (human) fatty tissues.

In contrast to these normal tissue data, few measurements are available for malignant tumors. We usually assume the values of σ (tumors) to be similar to the conductivity of muscle, but probably with a wide scatter of values. Moreover, in a given tumor the conductivity is likely to vary from one point to another, depending on capillary density and the extent of areas of necrosis. In addition, interstitial heating may damage some structures (such as the capillaries [108]) and this may lead to a modification of the conductivity characteristics of the tumors *during* the hyperthermia treatment. In addition, conductivity increases with temperature (by about 2% per °C).

The importance of such inhomogeneity of the electrical conductivity throughout the target volume has already been stressed by Cetas et al. [25, 98]. These authors prepared a phantom with a central core of conductivity lower than the rest of the phantom. When studying a thermogram taken after heating, they observed that the currents tended to diverge around the lower conductivity core, resulting in a core heating of only one-fourth that of the higher conductivity phantom edges.

Another important parameter governing the distribution of SAR, which is of major importance in the case of interstitial hyperthermia, is the shape and size (mainly the diameter) of the implanted electrodes. In the early days of the technique, it was thought that two rows of implanted needle-shaped electrodes could be equated with the two planes of electrodes of a capacitive system, and thus it was thought that both systems deposited the power quite uniformly throughout the intervening tissues [98]. In fact, more precise studies, particularly by Mechling, Strohbehn et al. [89, 123], showed that the low frequency needle system deposits its energy in a small region about each electrode. Utilizing the classical Maxwell's equation for electromagnetic problems, these authors were able to demonstrate that the power density, i.e., the SAR, falls off very rapidly away from the electrodes. Actually the power falls off approximately *as* $1/r^2$ where r is the distance from the electrode [123]. Moreover, the smaller the diameter of the needle-shaped electrode, the higher the power density located in a small volume just around the electrode. Thus very small (less than 1 mm) electrodes should be avoided because of the possibility of small areas of intense heating in the immediate vicinity of the probes.

The SAR is obviously one of the main parameters we have to know in order to be able to attempt to predict the temperature distribution when utilizing resistive interstitial heating. Another important point we have to take into account is the *blood flow*, acting in living tissues as a very efficient cooling system. While in a medium devoid of any type of cooling, resistive diathermy heating will result in a continuous increase in temperature up to high values, in a living tissue perfused with blood at about 37 °C, a steady state temperature can be achieved when the quantity of heat carried away by the blood circulation is equal to the heat deposited by the electric currents. Recognition of this heat balance has led to the development of a number of mathematical models allowing the temperature distribution to be estimated, taking into account:

1. The local temperature rise above normal tissue temperature
2. The density of tissue and blood respectively
3. The specific heat of tissue and blood respectively
4. The time
5. The thermal conductivity of tissue
6. The volumetric blood flow rate per unit mass of tissue
7. The temperature of blood entering the region in the arterial system, for localized hyperthermia (core temperature)
8. The power per unit volume of tissue generated by metabolic processes (usually very small in relative terms)

A detailed formulation of this equation, according to Strohbehn [123] is:

$$\varrho_t c_t \frac{\partial T(r,t)}{\partial t} = \nabla\cdot(k\nabla T) - \varrho_t \varrho_b c_b m (T-T_b) + \varrho_t \mathrm{SAR}(r,t) \qquad (1.1)$$

where k = thermal conductivity of tissue; ϱ_t, ϱ_b = density of tissue and blood, respectively; c_t, c_b = specific heat of tissue and blood, respectively; t = time; m = volumetric blood flow rate per unit mass of tissue; T = temperature; T_b = temperature of arterial blood entering the region, normally assumed to be at core temperature.

A more detailed account of the bioheat transfer equation can be found in [18, 19, 26, 56, 69, 74, 123]. This equation is known to have several limitations:

1. No description of "large" blood vessel effects
2. Lack of directionality
3. No distinction between tissue and blood temperatures
4. It takes no account of possible changes of the blood perfusion during an efficient hyperthermia treatment

It has, however, proved useful at least for the understanding of the temperature distribution patterns and of the respective roles of the various involved parameters.

Computer simulations based on the bioheat equation allowed Strohbehn et al. to demonstrate that the role of blood flow during resistive interstitial hyperthermia was of major importance. Strohbehn [121] calculated the isotherms for a ten-needle implantation (two planes of five needles), the spacing being 1 cm between each probe and between the two rows of five needles. The blood flow being equal to 0 and the maximum allowed temperature in this computer simulation being 45 °C, the "therapeutic" region largely encompasses the needle area and the heating is relatively homogeneous. If blood flow is chosen as being 2.7 ml/100 g min, and then 27 ml/100 g min, the distortion of the isotherms is striking. With a 27 ml/100 g min blood perfusion, at no point can we reach 45 °C; moreover, the total volume reaching at least 42.5 °C (the "therapeutic" volume according to Strohbehn's definition), is far smaller than without any blood flow, and hot areas are concentrated around the probes in spite of the short spacing. Other simulations with larger spacing of the electrodes predicted the total inability of the technique to heat in an acceptable way when blood flow reaches the value of 27 ml/100 g min. We must underline that the blood flow values chosen by Strohbehn are within the physiological range; the blood perfusion rate for resting muscle is about 2.7 ml/100 g min, and is much higher for active muscle. The value of 27 ml/100 g min is about a factor of 2 less than blood flow rates in normal brain [121]. Clearly, such computer models have their limitations. Firstly because of the limitations of the bioheat transfer equation itself (vide supra), and secondly because the computer models are generally two-dimensional, assuming the electrodes are infinitely long. The results should not be interpreted as providing an exact prediction of the temperature distribution, but they are useful to understand the patterns of resistive interstitial heating and to avoid major mistakes of implantation.

Actually, these physical studies allowed practical conclusions to be drawn that are of direct use both to the engineer who has to design a low frequency amplifier for interstitial heating, and to the clinician who has to implant a given tumor.

For the engineer, simple calculations based on the previously studied equations have shown that to reach a "therapeutic" heating, the machine must provide in the tumor a current density of approximately $15\ \mathrm{mA\ cm^{-2}}$, and a power density (ARD) of about $35\ \mathrm{mW\ cm^{-3}}$ [29]. Moreover, the now well-established inhomogeneity of several tissue parameters such as conductivity and blood perfusion must direct the engineers to design devices which are able to adapt the power in each implanted probe.

For the clinician the *diameter* of the implanted material (needles or tubes) must be in the range 1 – 1.6 mm. A smaller diameter would lead to unacceptable "hot spots" immediately around the probes, while a larger diameter would be uncomfortable for the patient. The optimal calculated *spacing of the electrodes* should be in the range 1 – 1.5 cm [125]. This is in good agreement with some early clinical data [31, 53].

Moreover, the study of the distribution of SAR emphasized the need for good implant geometry. In the case of two nonparallel electrodes, most of the power will concentrate in the area where the probes are closer, leading to an unacceptable distribution of temperature [36, 123]. For the same reason, the two electrodes of a pair should be of nearly *equal length*: if they are not one will observe a concentration of the power around the shortest probe, with once more a high risk of an unacceptable hot spot in this area [36]. In addition, the clinician must be aware of the fact that, when working at such low frequencies, good electrical contact between the metallic probes and the tissues is mandatory. A simple coating of the electrode by a plastic catheter or by some type of varnish provides complete insulation.

1.2.1.2 Technological Aspects

In the first clinical trials very simple "homemade" amplifiers were connected to two rows of implanted needles as initially proposed by Doss et al. [46]. In this system the same voltage was applied to all the needles in a given plane [31, 45]. It very soon appeared from physical (vide supra) and clinical studies that it was desirable to have the capability to control the voltage to each needle or probe [123].

To solve this problem, different technical approaches have been proposed. The French groups utilize a commercially available amplifier derived from initial prototypes developed at the Institut Gustave-Roussy [31, 34]. This machine consists of three generators (25 W each) supplying three independent circuits. Each generator is connected to a pair of implanted electrodes. The frequency of each pair can be chosen to be the same or slightly different, in a range of 0.5–1 MHz. A different frequency for each pair avoids most interference and makes the regulation of the machine easier. The power applied to each of the six lines can be adjusted individually. The generator is connected to needle-shaped probes able to transmit the power to the implanted material. Each needle-shaped probe is equipped with thermistors for temperature recording (it was checked that there was no interference between the thermistors and the generator in this frequency range) and for power adjustment to preset temperatures. Each heating line is equipped with an individual and adjustable safety device to prevent the temperature from exceeding a preset temperature (usually 46 °C).

In a recently updated version of the machine, a computer program permits the recording of clinical and thermometric data for each hyperthermia treatment. Since the number of available probes (now up to eight) is relatively small, most of the groups are now working with two or three units, connected together, in order to allow large multiple needle implantations [35, 37].

In parallel, Astrahan et al. [5, 6] proposed another solution, which also gave birth to a commercially available unit. The basic concept was to "time share" the same voltage between the pairs of electrodes. In this system a powerful amplifier (300 W) is connected to up to 20 pairs of electrodes. A multiplexer switches the voltage sequentially from one pair of electrodes to the next, the total sequencing time not exceeding 5 s. The sequencing parameters of time and order of connection are programmable from a computer keyboard. This makes possible empirical modifications of the temperature distributions by varying the relative duty cycle of each needle pair. The present unit also allows an automatic regulation by feedback from one or several additionally implanted thermocouples. Thermometric data from up to 15 measurement points are directly and continuously available on the computer screen. The program also allows clear recording of all clinical and thermometric data [78].

The flexibility of these two systems usually allows the clinician, after some automatic or manual adjustments, to achieve homogeneous heating within the volume which is encompassed by the implanted electrodes. However, some (rare) situations remain problematical. For example, a potential problem for both the above alternatives is that one of the needles in a pair could be hotter than desired while the other is too cold. Adjustment of the power, changing the polarity and/or the frequency, does not always solve this problem, which is more likely to happen if the spacing of the electrodes is rather large, if the two electrodes of a pair are located in two different conductivity mediums, or if one electrode of a pair has been implanted rather close to a large vessel.

Hence a third alternative is being developed at Stanford University by Prionas et al. [103, 123]. In a search for a rational procedure to decide which electrodes should be connected together and for how long, these authors developed a sophisticated computer-assisted system able to connect the two coolest electrodes together. This new machine is presently being tested clinically.

Although the description of the implantation material is part of the technology, this particular aspect will be extensively described in Sect. 1.2.5.1 and the following clinical section when considering the various techniques of implantation.

1.2.2 Radiative Microwave Interstitial Heating

1.2.2.1 Physical Aspects

The basic physical concepts of radiative interstitial heating are completely different from those which govern resistive heating [47, 123]. This alternative technique utilizes a radiative antenna usually working in a range 300–2450 MHz. Although the design of the antennae varies among the different groups, a classical – simplified – feature is shown in Fig. 1.1. The antenna consists of a coaxial probe: at the tip of

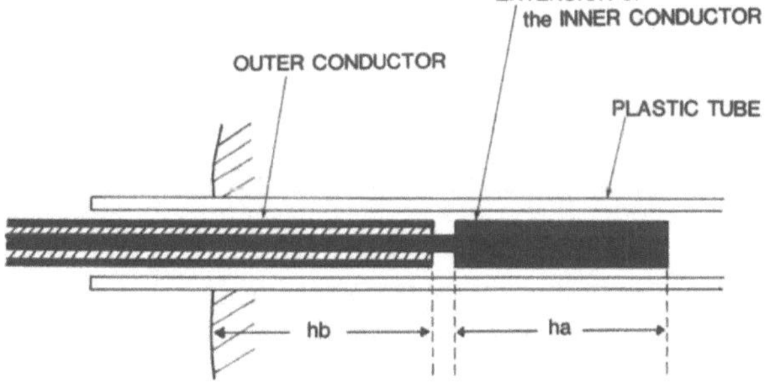

Fig. 1.1. Classical bipolar microwave antenna [75, 123]

the probe the inner conductor is usually extended, forming the final section of the antenna, denoted by *ha* in Fig. 1.1 (according to [123]). The outer conductor forms the proximal part, denoted by *hb*. The voltage at the gap between the two sections *ha* and *hb* produces a current that flows away from the junction, creating an electromagnetic wave propagating as a "water wave propagates away from a pebble dropped into a pond" [123]. This type of antenna is denoted as a bipolar [75] or dipole [123] antenna. It has been shown, both theoretically and experimentally, that the antennae perform best if $ha = hb$ [123].

While in the previously considered RF technique a very thin layer of insulation completely stops the currents, in this microwave radiating technique it can be shown (both theoretically and practically) that a layer of insulation located between the antenna and the tissue *improves* the way the antenna radiates [123].

Another important difference from the RF procedure is that in the case of radiative heating, the *choice of frequency* is of major importance. The bipolar or dipole antennae tend to radiate better if the length of the implanted probe is a half wavelength in the composite medium "antenna-insulation layer-surrounding tissues". Thus the length of the antenna should theoretically be about 18 cm at 300 MHz, about 7 cm at 915 MHz (the most commonly utilized length), and about 2.5 cm at 2450 MHz (not really convenient in the clinic).

So far we have only considered the patterns of heating for one isolated probe. Since a "typical" microwave antenna can only heat a volume which is grossly in the shape of an elongated ellipsoid of revolution of about 2 cm in the radial direction and about 5–6 cm in the longitudinal direction (at 915 MHz), we obviously have to implant *arrays* of antennae in the clinical situation. Either a *coherent* or an *incoherent* system can be chosen. In an incoherent system each antenna is acting independently while in a coherent system the distribution of power density (SAR) depends on the phasing between the implanted antennae, which gives rise to constructive or destructive interferences.

Actually in the radiative system, most of the parameters governing the distribution of the SAR are related to the design of the antennae: (a) relative length of the inner and outer conductors, (b) total length of these two sections (depending on the frequency), (c) type of insulation, and (d) choice of a coherent or of an incoherent mode. But some parameters, directly related to the implanted medium – such as electrical characteristics – probably also play a role in the distribution of power density (SAR). These parameters perhaps explain some discrepancies which have been observed between theoretical calculations and experimental measurements. For example, theoretical computations at the junction plane of four radiating antennae working in a coherent mode predict that the maximum SAR is *at the center* of the implantation, and *greater* than at the antennae. However, experimental measurements have shown that, if it is true that some kind of hot spot is seen at the center of the array, it is only about 80% of the maximum at one of the antennae [123]. These discrepancies between computer-predicted and measured values could also be explained by some technological problems: antennae and cables have to be matched very carefully. Moreover, as previously shown in Sect. 1.2.1, the blood flow remains a major parameter when considering not only the distribution of SAR but also the final distribution of temperatures [123, 125].

Finally, these physical aspects raise important questions for the engineers. The first is the question of the length of the antennae: a classical amplifier working at 915 MHz can only supply 7-cm antennae only able to efficiently heat about 5 cm. This lack of adjustability of the length of the antennae is obviously a major drawback for the clinician. The second problem is the shape of the isotherms (or iso-SAR curves) around a given probe. Although the theory predicts the shape on an (American) football or of an elongated ellipsoid of revolution (which is already a serious limitation for the clinician), in fact most measurements show "pear-shaped" distribution curves. The last problem is that of the choice between the coherent and incoherent mode of working. In the incoherent system each antenna acts independently, and the regulation is easier. The coherent system is appealing since in can create hot spots in specifically located points, but the precise control of these hot spots remains somewhat problematical.

1.2.2.2 Technological Aspects

Several systems are presently commercially available for microwave interstitial heating, but not all the technological problems have been solved.

To avoid the irregular shape of the iso-SAR curves around the radiative antennae, and to achieve good uniformity of the dissipated power along the probe, use of a tapered dielectric coating has been proposed [75]. However, such a coating could impair the introduction of the antennae into the classical plastic carriers usually utilized for the implantation. Other efforts are underway to find means of obtaining better heating toward the tips of the antennae [110].

One of the major remaining problems is that of the length of effective heating when working with radiative probes. One solution is to have available an amplifier able to provide different frequencies (from 300 to 2450 MHz) and thus to supply antennae of various lengths, so that the clinician can adapt the heating probes to the size and the shape of the tumor. Although possible, this technique is rather complicated. Moreover, since an irregularly shaped tumor can force the clinician to use antennae of very different lengths, the frequencies of the antennae must be different, rendering impossible heating in a coherent mode. So different research groups are presently looking at modifications of the antennae so that it is possible to adjust the length of the SAR patterns *without changing* the frequency of the generator [43, 62, 123].

For example, an interesting modification of the classical microwave antenna was recently reported by Lee et al. [76]. These authors removed sections of the outer conductor, thus creating additional junctions, or "nodes." In their experience, a 3-cm outer conductor segment worked best for a two-junction applicator, and 2-cm outer conductor segments for a three-junction applicator (in this case, the classical outer conductor plus two segments). A 1-cm gap between the segments was chosen. Precise measurements of both isotherms (in steady state phantoms) and of SAR showed a marked improvement of the treated volume and of the homogeneity of heating around the probe. It is worth noting that attempts to produce an applicator with more than three junctions were unsuccessful. This new device has not yet been tested clinically.

The last problem is the difficult choice between the incoherent and coherent systems. We previously saw that each system has its advantages and drawbacks. It would obviously be desirable to *combine* the advantages of both modes. Strohbehn and Douple [122, 127] have described such an attempt. Their microwave power source generates 300 W at 915 MHz. The system turns all the antennae on at the beginning of a 1-s cycle and is at that time operating in a coherent mode. However, each antenna is turned off at a different time, depending on the average power needed to keep that antenna at the correct preset temperature (due to a feedback system, based on fiberoptic temperature probes inserted in the implanted catheters with the antennae and connected to a computer). Clearly, once the antennae start to turn off independently the value of the coherency is lost.

Finally, the systems presently available commercially still have some limitations, essentially due to the fact that the distribution of the SAR is extremely sensitive to small changes in the antennae parameters. We can reasonably hope that more satisfactory designs will be forthcoming soon.

1.2.3 Inductively Heated Ferromagnetic Seeds

This third alternative technique for interstitial hyperthermia is being developed in two American centers: the University of Arizona Medical Center in Tucson [42, 59, 80, 87, 120] and the University of Alabama in Birmingham [7, 21]. The technique consists of the implantation of a totally passive device; ferromagnetic seeds or needles that can be selectively heated by an external power source. After the implantation of an array of such a material, the patient (so far only the phantom or the animal) is placed in a concentric coil energized by an alternating current, usually in the 0.5 – 2 MHz range. This current produces a magnetic field in the axial direction of the patient, which creates eddy currents both in the tissues and in the ferromagnetic implanted material. The frequency must be chosen so that the absorbed power density per cm^3 of tumor (from the seeds or needles) should be significantly higher than the absorbed power density per cm^3 normal tissue. This problem was studied by Stauffer et al. [120] and it was concluded that the operating frequency should be below 0.5 MHz. However, other studies by Wait [140] suggested that not all the necessary parameters were taken into account for this calculation.

The main problem which arose with this system is the control of temperature. Not only did the temperature have to be measured by some kind of implanted thermometer, but the applied power produced a continuous increase of the temperature in the seeds – or needles – possibly up to unacceptably high values. In order to overcome this problem, the Arizona and Alabama groups developed newly designed seeds made of a composite material whose curie point was about 45 °– 47 °C. Thus, when reaching this temperature, the magnetic properties of the alloy change, and the implanted material is no longer heated. These new seeds (for example of a nickel-copper alloy) are thus able to self-regulate their maximum temperature.

One of the main differences between the ferromagnetic seed procedure and the two previously described interstitial hyperthermia techniques is that in both resistive and radiative interstitial procedures the power is deposited within the tissues, whereas with the ferromagnetic seed technique the power is only deposited in the seeds and one must rely solely on heat conduction to smooth out the temperature distributions.

The temperature patterns throughout the implanted tumor are closely dependent on the size of the material (usually about 1 mm in diameter) and on the geometry of the implantation. These parameters were dis-

cussed by Stauffer et al. [120] and Wait [140]. When using the bioheat transfer equation [123] it is clear that this system is highly sensitive to blood flow variation within the tumor [89]. Brezovich et al. [21] and Matloubieh et al. [87] were able to calculate that this technique can lead to acceptably uniform temperature distributions throughout a tumor with a *low* blood flow, whereas it appears impossible to achieve homogeneous heating in a given tumor with a high blood flow, due to cold spots between the seeds, even if these seeds have been implanted quite close together.
In conclusion, this technique clearly has its limitations, but it is younger than the two previously studied ones, and one can expect further refinements.

1.2.4 Other Techniques

We shall consider here some techniques which cannot be really referred to as "classical" radiofrequency or microwave interstitial procedures. The common feature of these techniques is that they utilize the currents flowing between an implanted material (thus really "interstitial") and different types of "external" (or intracavitary) electrode.
The first group who reported such an attempt was again from Tucson [82]. Manning et al. reported the treatment of a paravaginal tumor using two rows of implanted needles (working exactly in the way described in Sect. 1.2.1), but also using a row of needles located *at the surface* of a plastic vaginal applicator, in contact with the vaginal mucosa. This technique is actually very similar to the "classical" low frequency technique, provided that the spacing between the external (here intracavitary) row and the implanted needles remains in the usual range. The clinical results have proved to be approximately the same as for the classical radiofrequency technique. Similar procedures have been extensively utilized by Syed, who designed special applicators for pelvic implantations. The vaginal part of one of these sophisticated templates has been prepared so that it can receive several needles at its surface (with a 1 cm spacing) [129–131]. The groups at Tucson, Lyon, Villejuif, and elsewhere have also used this type of template [37, 82]. There are other types of applicator available which can be used in a similar way, such as that designed by Martinez et al. [85, 86].
The group from Birmingham proposed a rather different approach. Their technique is based on the currents flowing between various types of implanted electrode and large external plates. After theoretical studies, several experiments were performed on phantoms. They studied the heating patterns which were obtained when working with an array of implanted needles (the "internal" conductor) and a outer metallic cylinder (the "external" conductor), a 1.5 MHz frequency power being applied between both electrodes. With satisfactory results [77], Lilly et al. then studied the possibility of heating using an internal coil of 18 gauge stainless steel, inserted as a corkscrew in a rat experimental tumor. The whole animal (except the head) was placed in a 0.44% NaCl bath at 37 °C. The external conductor consisted of a screen wire cage surrounding the rat trunk (and tumor). The applied frequency was 13.56 MHz. Again, the temperature profiles which were obtained were encouraging. To date, they have reported only one case of such a treatment in a patient. A temperature of 42 °C could be achieved in the tumor (an unresectable pulmonary carcinoma), but the patient died rapidly from complications unrelated to hyperthermia [22].
A different technique is currently under study by the group from Nancy, France (Marchal et al. [83]). These authors developed an original adaptation of the classical radiative technique. They do not use a bipolar antenna but a simple "monopole" antenna, the "outer conductor" being in this case constituted by the patient himself. It works at a frequency of 27 MHz. A major advantage of the technique is that it allows the use on any length of antenna up to 15 and possibly 20 cm. After theoretical calculations and experiments in phantoms, five patients were treated. Since in Nancy the usual spacing between the tubes is about 2–2.5 cm, the temperature distribution (as predicted by the previous theoretical calculations) was not found to be satisfactory. Further refinements of the apparatus and slight modifications of the technique of brachytherapy implantation are being studied.
In parallel, after contacts with the Nancy group, Visser et al. developed a similar technique in Rotterdam. The preliminary results they obtained in phantoms, then in animals, are obviously encouraging [137].
This new technique could overcome one of the problems still unsolved in microwave interstitial hyperthermia: the need for an easy adaptation of the length of the heating antennae.

1.2.5 Comparative Study of the Different Techniques for Interstitial Hyperthermia

If we consider in detail the two main interstitial heating procedures, the radiofrequency resistive heating

and the microwave radiative techniques, we observe that both can be safe and effective in experienced hands [28, 36]. However, they have different advantages and disadvantages. The relative merits of each interstitial hyperthermia system must be considered, with particular regard to compatibility with brachytherapy systems (which vary a little in each institution). We must not forget in this discussion that interstitial hyperthermia is no longer used alone, but always combined with brachytherapy.
The following will be considered:

1. The material for implantation
2. The number of implanted electrodes
3. The spacing of the probes
4. The length of the electrodes
5. The distribution of temperature around the probes
6. The thermometry

1.2.5.1 Material for the Implantations

There is no major problem for the brachytherapists using the microwave radiative technique. We previously saw that the presence of a layer of insulation was not only possible, but advisable. Thus the classical plastic tubes currently employed for most brachytherapy implantations also can be utilized here. The microwave antennae radiate through the tubes (see Sect. 1.2.2) without any problems.
The situation is entirely different for the radiofrequency resistive technique: in that case good electrical contact between a metallic probe and the tissues is essential. The classical plastic tubes of curietherapy would act here as complete insulators, preventing any current from flowing between the electrodes. The first clinical implantations were performed using metallic needles, but the drawbacks of such a material soon became obvious. Firstly these rigid needles were uncomfortable for the patients during the 2–5 days necessary for the brachytherapy application. Secondly, the metallic needles were heating all along their length; very often a significant volume of healthy tissues was unnecessarily heated together with the tumor. In addition, blisters were sometimes noted at the entry and exit points of the needles [72, 78].
To overcome this last problem, all the groups utilizing resistive heating developed some type of insulation for the parts of the needles passing through the normal tissues and the skin. Complete insulation could be easily achieved either by means of a plastic catheter overcoating the metallic needle, or by "painting" the desired part of the needle with a varnish, or by partially shielding the metallic material with "heat-shrink" polyolefin tubing [77]. All these solutions were convenient for some implants, but they did not solve the problem of the rigidity and the discomfort of the metallic implants. Two solutions were proposed: The Villejuif group designed special plastic tubes, with a metallic portion centered away from the ends (the three parts being simply glued together). The metallic length, that is to say the "heating" length, can be individualized for each implantation. The external diameter of both plastic and metallic tubes is 1.6 mm. The power is brought to the metallic part from the amplifier by means of a metallic probe which is pushed into the plastic end of the tube until it contacts the metallic part [31, 32] (Fig. 1.2). More recently the Stanford group (Prionas et al. [103]) developed completely flexible plastic tubes with a thin

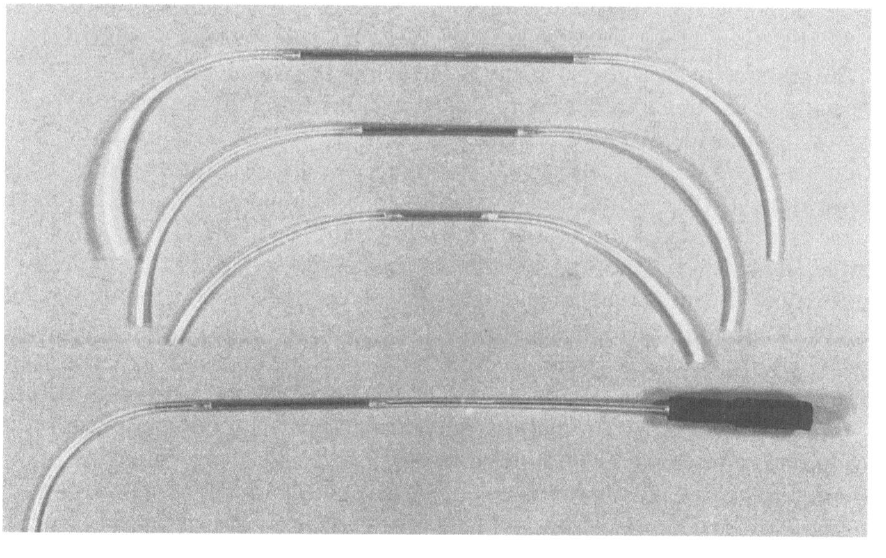

Fig. 1.2. The metal–plastic tubes used by the group in Villejuif (France) for radiofrequency interstitial heating. *Below* : connection of the amplifier probe

layer of metal coating, whose length can be customized for the particular tumor to be heated.
Actually, we shall see later that the choice of either solution (insulation coating of metallic probes), or more sophisticated "metal – plastic" tubes) closely depends on the type of implantation to be performed.

1.2.5.2 Number of Implanted Electrodes

Here again, the situation is simple with the microwave radiative technique. The number of probes is not limited (if working in a noncoherent system). It is only dictated by the number of the available electrodes of a given machine.
When using radiofrequency resistive heating, an even number of implanted probes is theoretically required since, as previously stated, the currents flow between *pairs* of electrodes. This can be a limitation for the brachytherapist who is not used to being concerned whether odd or even numbers of implanted probes are required. It is clearly advisable to implant an even number of electrodes. However, with the more sophisticated machines available (see Sect. 1.2.1.2) it is possible to achieve satisfactory heating with an odd number of probes, although the regulation of the power in each probe of such a system is obviously more difficult in this unusual situation.

1.2.5.3 Spacing of the Probes

For the radiofrequency resistive technique, the theoretical predictions, particularly by Mechling and Strohbehn [89, 121], agree with the clinical observations that the needle spacing should not exceed 1.5 cm to avoid large temperature gradients in the heated volume. The optimal compromise value for the spacing of the implanted electrodes appears to be 1.2 – 1.3 mm. In fact, this is in the range of the usual spacing of the implanted tubes for brachytherapy implants using iridium 192 wires [101].
Some authors working with the microwave technique have claimed that a major advantage of this procedure is that the spacing of the electrodes could be larger than 1.5 cm (the upper limit for the previous technique). If this is theoretically true [89], it has not always been confirmed clinically, and it does not appear wise to advise a spacing of the probes in the range 2 – 2.5 cm.
Moreover, we must not forget that interstitial hyperthermia is always used with brachytherapy. This irradiation technique must govern, to some extent, the geometry of the implantation. A 2.5 cm spacing between the iridium 192 wires leads to areas of overdose around the radioactive material. Hence, even if theoretically the spacing of the probes could be a little larger with the radiative technique than with the resistive one, the inevitable association with brachytherapy makes a spacing in the range 1 – 1.5 cm advisable for both techniques [89].

1.2.5.4 Length of the Electrodes

For this problem the radiofrequency resistive technique clearly has advantages at least at the present time.
We previously noted that it is simple to adapt the effective heating length to a particular tumor, either by means of insulating some parts of metallic probes or by employing the more sophisticated tubes developed in Villejuif or Stanford [31, 103].
The problem is more complex with the microwave radiative technique, since the effective heating length depends on the frequency and on the precise design of the antennae. Most antennae which have been used up to now have been in the range 6 – 7 cm. At present the flexibility of this technique (for the problem of the electrode length) has not reached that of the resistive procedure. As previously stated, several groups are presently working on antennae in which the length of SAR pattern can be varied without changing the frequency of the generator. This would be a major step forward for the radiative technique.

1.2.5.5 Distribution of the Temperature Around the Probes

The distribution of the temperature around the implanted probes, in the direction of the axis of the implanted electrodes, will now be discussed in more depth.
In the resistive technique, it has been shown, both theoretically and clinically, that the distribution of temperature along the probe, and just around it, is most often quite homogeneous (except at the very end of the electrodes, where the temperature falls off). The isotherms immediately adjacent to the probe adapt the shape of a regular cylinder. The only exceptions are probably when a long needle is passing through tissues of very different conductivities, or when a part of a needle is located very close to a large vessel.
The distribution of the isotherms around the microwave antennae in the radiative technique is quite different. For a typical antenna the shape of the closer isotherms is like that of an American football or of an

elongated ellipsoid of revolution, and is sometimes more irregular, depending on the characteristics of the antenna [123]. The introduction of additional junctions (Lee et al. [76]) seems to improve the quality of heating around the probe.

In order to make this distribution of temperature less variable around the axis of the antennae, some groups proposed "tapering" the insulation layer around the radiative probe [75]. But this problem has not yet found an entirely satisfactory solution.

Recently, Mechling and Strohbehn [89] published a theoretical comparison of the temperature distributions produced by three interstitial hyperthermia systems, RF, microwaves, and ferromagnetic seeds. The results clearly depend on the spacing of the implanted heating probes and on the normal tissue and tumor blood flow simulation. The authors defined a hyperthermia equipment performance (HEP) rating as a criterion for comparing the various systems. The ferromagnetic seeds HEP was the least satisfactory in almost all the tested conditions. On the other hand, comparison of RF and microwaves showed that with a 1 cm implant spacing the RF needles heated about the same amount as the microwave antennae. With a 2 or 3 cm implant spacing the microwave antennae heated better than the RF needles. Since the basic spacing is in fact determined by the brachytherapy considerations and since the usual brachytherapy spacing is close to 1 cm, this means that in the usual situations the temperature distributions achieved by RF and microwave are grossly superimposable [89].

1.2.5.6 Thermometry

When working with radiofrequencies (in the range of 0.5 – 1 MHz), any type of thermometer can be utilized. We know that there is no interference between those 0.5 – 1 MHz resistive currents and the "classical" thermometers such as ordinary thermistors or thermocouples. This absence of interference has been confirmed several times clinically by different groups [31, 77]. Thus cheap "classical" thermistors and/or thermocouples can be utilized without any limitation in a volume heated by a radiofrequency resistive system.

The situation is different when working with microwaves in the usual range of 915 – 2450 MHz, in which case the thermocouple and thermistor probes are subject to perturbational interferences from the electromagnetic field. This perturbation can be minimized by orientating the thermometric probes so that they lie perpendicular to the microwave antennae, but this type of geometry for the implantation is usually highly impractical: most of the time, the catheters run parallel to one another in a "classical" implant. Another way of avoiding this problem is to switch off the power before each temperature reading. As shown in Fig. 1.3, we first observe a sharp temperature drop (a), corresponding to the perturbing interferences, then a slower decay (b). The usual procedure is to record the temperature at the breakpoint of the temperature curve. However, it is perhaps more precise to extrapolate back to time 0 to take into account the interruption of power input (Fig. 1.3). This technique needs thermometers that do not self-heat (i.e., well-insulated thermometers) and a very fast reading of the temperature after the power has been switched off (half a second?). This solution is in fact not very convenient and highly time consuming if complete thermal mapping is to be obtained throughout the whole hyperthermia session.

Clinicians using the microwave radiative technique now resort to specially designed noninterferent thermistors (high resistive thermistors with carbon-impregnated plastic leads) or to fiberoptic probes (fiberoptic leads and gallium arsenide sensors) so that temperature readings are not perturbed by the surrounding electromagnetic field. The only problem is the cost of this thermometric equipment, the fiberoptic thermometers being far more expansive than the ordinary thermocouples or thermistors.

Recently, Yerushalmi et al. designed a filtered thermocouple connected to a computer (for automatic correction of the remaining error after filtration). This new device is presently being studied in several centers [144].

Table 1.1 summarizes the respective advantages and drawbacks of resistive and radiative interstitial diathermy techniques.

Returning briefly to ferromagnetic seed techniques, several advantages can be found: (a) once the implantation has been performed, several hyperthermia sessions can be given very simply; (b) the self-regulating seeds guarantee the maximum possible temperature in the implanted material; (c) the small seeds (some millimeters) can be inserted in locations where the implantation of the classical plastic carriers is difficult. For example, good results were obtained in dogs presenting with a tumor destroying the facial bones, an area where the tube technique would probably have been impossible.

On the other hand there are some clear drawbacks. Unless the developments of noninvasive thermometry soon allow the clinician to obtain detailed thermal mapping without any thermometer implantation, we will still have to insert catheters to record the tumor temperature between the seeds. It is quite impossible

Table 1.1 Advantages and disadvantages of resistive and radiative interstitial diathermy techniques

	Radiofrequency resistive technique	Microwave radiative technique
Material for implantation	Metallic needles Special "metal-plastic" tubes	Usual plastic tubes used for brachytherapy applications
Number of implanted electrodes	Even	No theoretical limitation
Spacing of the probes	1 – 1.5 cm	Up to 2 cm (1.5 cm advisable)
Length of the heating	No theoretical limitation	Depends on the antenna design and on the *frequency*
Distribution of temperature around the probes	Regular cylindrical shape	Ellipsoid of revolution and sometimes pear shape
Thermometry	No limitation	Perturbs the usual thermistors and thermocouples Fiberoptic thermometric probes advisable

to predict this temperature theoretically. We previously noted that the seed technique was highly sensitive to blood flow, a parameter that we cannot assess precisely enough at the present time for a given tumor. Another drawback is the lack of "flexibility" once the implantation is performed. With the resistive or the radiative techniques, one can regulate the power in each heating probe. With the ferromagnetic seeds, if the geometry proves unsatisfactory, there is no way to "correct" the problem and to achieve homogeneous heating.
As previously stated, further refinements of this technique are awaited before drawing definitive conclusions.

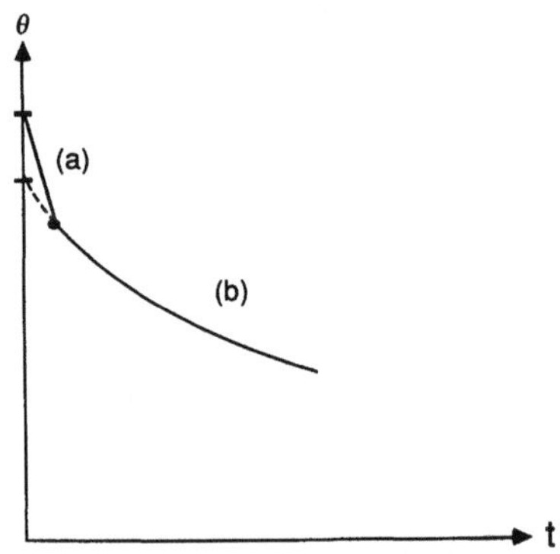

Fig. 1.3. Temperature decay of ordinary thermocouples or thermistors in a perturbing field. θ, temperature; t time

1.3 Clinical Aspects of Interstitial Hyperthermia

1.3.1 Techniques of Implantation

1.3.1.1 Anesthesia

While general anesthesia is the ideal method for both patient comfort and the ease of the operator performing the implant, this may be contraindicated in many patients who are considered for interstitial hyperthermia either because of age, poor general condition, or both. At Villejuif there is considerable experience in the use of a combination of light sedation and local anesthesia for patients with superficially accessible lesions of limited size [34]. Joseph et al. used the same procedure for some patients [72]. It is safe and well tolerated, provided precise rules are obeyed. Only the preplanned channels of the needles are carefully locally anesthetized. This allows an implantation of the needles without any pain and limits the amount of local anesthetics utilized.
The techniques of implantation closely depend on the anatomical sites and on the tumor morphology (size and shape). We will discuss the various possible techniques for three principal sites:

1. Superficial lesions
2. Head and neck tumors
3. Pelvic tumors

1.3.1.2 Techniques of Implantation for Superficial Lesions

When using a *radiofrequency heating procedure*, very precise pretreatment planning is warranted. The following are the principal parameters of the implant which should be decided *before* the procedure:

1. Number of probes
2. Length of the heating parts of the probes (or length of the volume to be heated)
3. Number of planes
4. Geometry of the implant
5. Location of entry and exit points

The *number of probes* depends on the size of the tumor. The spacing of the electrodes must remain in the range 1 – 1.5 cm. It is usual and preferable to work with an even number of probes.

The *length of the heating parts* of the probes (metallic parts of the special "hyperthermia" tubes or noninsulated parts of ordinary metallic needles) depends on the tumor size and on the necessary "safety margin" which must be treated around the tumor. It is advisable for the heated volume to encompass the tumor itself with a generous margin (of at least 2 cm if possible).

The *number of planes*, or of rows of probes, depends in those superficial lesions on the thickness of the tumor. The spacing between the planes should be the same (or about the same) as that between the probes in a given plane. Any number of planes can be utilized: we partly disagree with Strohbehn [123] when he suggests that a single plane geometry is "not effective for low-frequency electrodes." Figure 1.4 shows different possibilities of connection for one-, two-, or three-plane implants. However, we agree with the point that this monoplanar technique can only heat a thin layer. This will be further specified.

The *geometry* should be as perfect as possible. The *parallelism* of the probes is of paramount importance. Even slightly converging electrodes can lead to an unacceptable inhomogeneity of the temperature distribution, with hot and/or cold spots within the treated volume [36, 123]. The best solution to ensure good geometry is to maintain the outer parts of the tubes or needles with some type of rigid preperforated material which acts as a template immobilization device (e.g., plastic templates or additional preperforated plastic tubes – see below).

The *location of the entry and exit points* depends on the size of the tumor, on the length of the heating parts of the implanted material, and on the insulated length under the skin. It seems advisable to leave at least 1 – 1.5 cm of insulation at each end between the metallic heating part and both the entry and exit points of the implanted material through the skin (see Fig. 1.5 for a schematic diagram of a four-probe implant).

Thus before the implantation begins, very precise marks are drawn on the skin of the patients, indicating the planned entry and exit points of the implantation material, the skin projection of the tumor, and the projection of the needles or tubes to be implanted. If necessary, this preimplantation drawing will be discussed with an experienced brachytherapist to ensure that the proposed implant geometry is also suitable for effective brachytherapy.

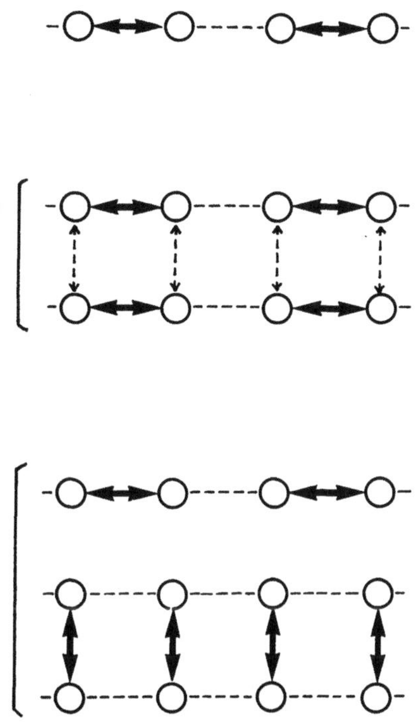

Fig. 1.4. RF technique. Possible connections of the probes for one-, two- or three-plane implants

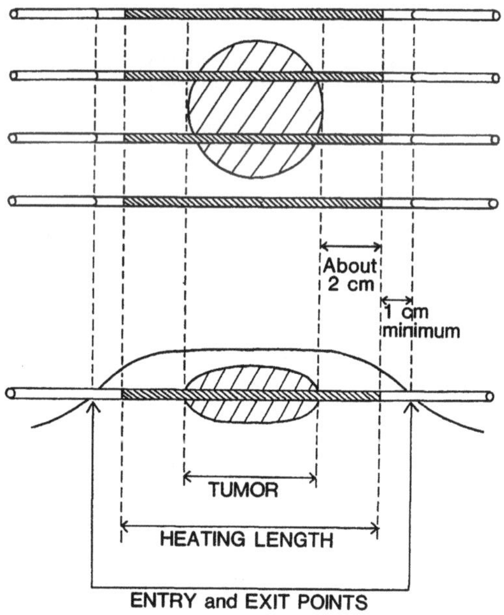

Fig. 1.5. RF technique. Schematic diagram of a four-probe implant

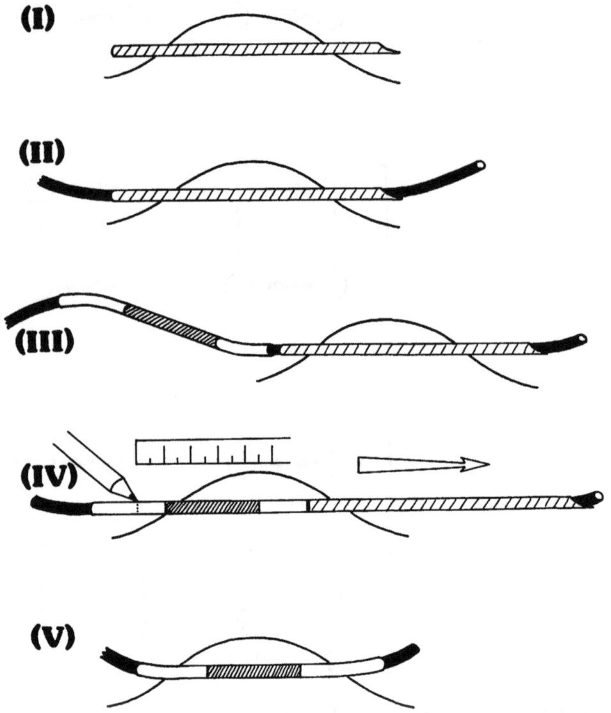

Fig. 1.6. Successive steps of the implantation of a metal–plastic hyperthermia tube for RF heating. *I*, Implantation of a metallic needle. *II*, Insertion of a nylon wire guide through the needle. *III*, Placement of the hyperthermia tube over the nylon guide. *IV*, Removal of the metallic needle and placement of the hyperthermia tube. A pencil mark indicates the desired insulation length. *V*, Complete removal of the metallic needle. Definitive placement of the hyperthermia tube. Insertion of a lead wire to avoid kinking of the plastic parts

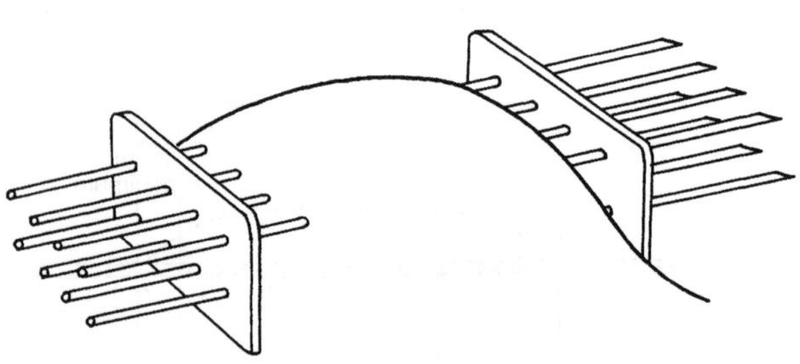

Fig. 1.7. Needle immobilization system by Plexiglas or plastic plates

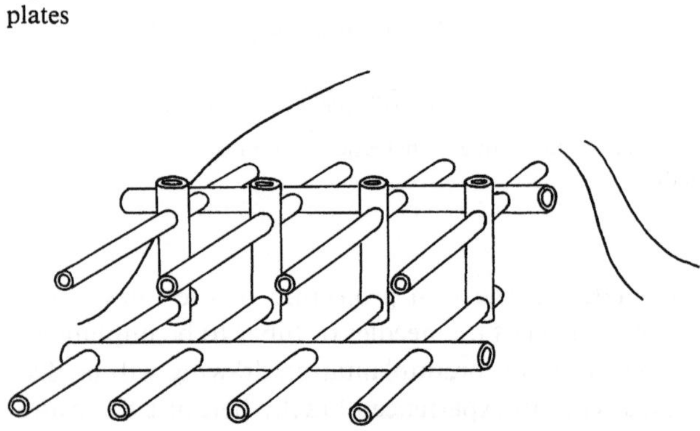

Fig. 1.8. Tube immobilization system by plastic tubes of a larger diameter

If using partly insulated *metallic needles*, these can be directly inserted according to the geometry which has been decided. Precise measurements are mandatory to ensure that the insulated parts correctly shield a 1 – 1.5 cm length from the skin entry point.
When using the special *"hyperthermia" tubes*, such as those designed by the Villejuif or Stanford group [31, 103], the method of implantation is that of the classical plastic carriers commonly used in brachytherapy, but with two differences. Firstly these sophisticated tubes are more fragile than the simple plastic ones and must be inserted with great care, in order to avoid any disconnection between the plastic and metallic parts. Secondly, as for the needles, very precise measurements are mandatory to make sure that the insulated length (in those cases the plastic parts) is located in the correct position. The details of the implantation of such a hyperthermia tube are shown in Fig. 1.6.
Once the material is implanted, it is usually useful to maintain the outer parts of the needles or of the tubes by some type of template immobilization device. This system has two roles: firstly it homogenizes the spacing between the probes, and secondly it makes sure that this spacing will stay constant throughout the treatment time (hyperthermia and brachytherapy). Without this immobilization, edema may collect (usually just after the implantation) and force apart the needles or the tubes, thus disturbing the implant geometry.
When metallic needles are used, essentially if two or more planes are implanted, the immobilization template system usually consists of preperforated Plexiglas or plastic plates, as shown in Fig. 1.7.
When the hyperthermia tubes are used, it seems more convenient to utilize perforated plastic tubes of a larger diameter, as shown in Fig. 1.8. The different planes of the same implantation can be linked together by the same plastic tube technique.
To avoid coagulation of blood remaining inside the needles or the tubes, heparin solution is immediately injected into each implanted probe.
If hyperthermia is not performed immediately after the implantation, a guide must be kept in the hyperthermia tubes to avoid the occlusion by blood which may occur in spite of heparin instillation and also to prevent any kinking of the plastic parts of the tubes. This guide can be a simple nylon wire, or a lead wire (which has the potential advantage of being visible on check radiographs). Additional "buttons" are also usually placed on the outer parts of the tubes to avoid any displacement of the implanted material. In the classical brachytherapy technique, these buttons are usually tightened around the tubes. For hyperthermia, it is not advisable to tighten the buttons too firmly,

since the subsequent insertion of the probe bringing the power from the generator can be rendered difficult.

The problem of the necessary number of implanted planes deserves further discussion. We previously assumed that it was possible, using a low frequency technique, to work with only one plane of needles or tubes, provided that we clearly recognize the limits of this technique.

With a "classical" 1.2 cm spacing, for example, it will only be possible to heat a thickness of a few millimeters (to be precisely measured with additionally implanted catheters). Moreover, the 85% reference isodose of the Paris system dosimetry will only encompass, at midpoint between the lines, a thickness of 0.6 cm [48].

In addition, the superficial millimeters are usually cooled by ambient air. Thus this kind of monoplanar implant can only be proposed for very superficial and thin lesions (roughly no more than 5 mm). Clinically this situation is found not infrequently. For example, chest wall recurrences of breast carcinomas often consist of small cutaneous nodules whose thickness is only a few millimeters (Fig. 1.9).

When the thickness of the tumor is over 0.5 cm, the best solution is without doubt to implant two rows of electrodes (one deep and one superficial, parallel to the skin surface) (Fig. 1.10). A difficult problem arises when the thickness of the lesion is about 0.6–0.9 cm, and when the deep plane is limited by an underlying organ which cannot be implanted (e.g., bone or artery). Here again a classical clinical situa-

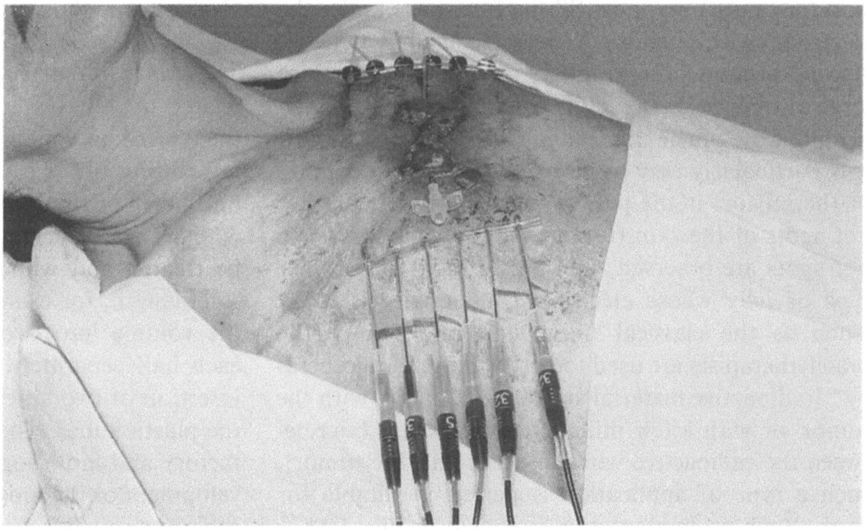

Fig. 1.9. Monoplanar implantation for a chest wall relapse of a breast cancer. RF technique with the Villejuif metal–plastic tubes

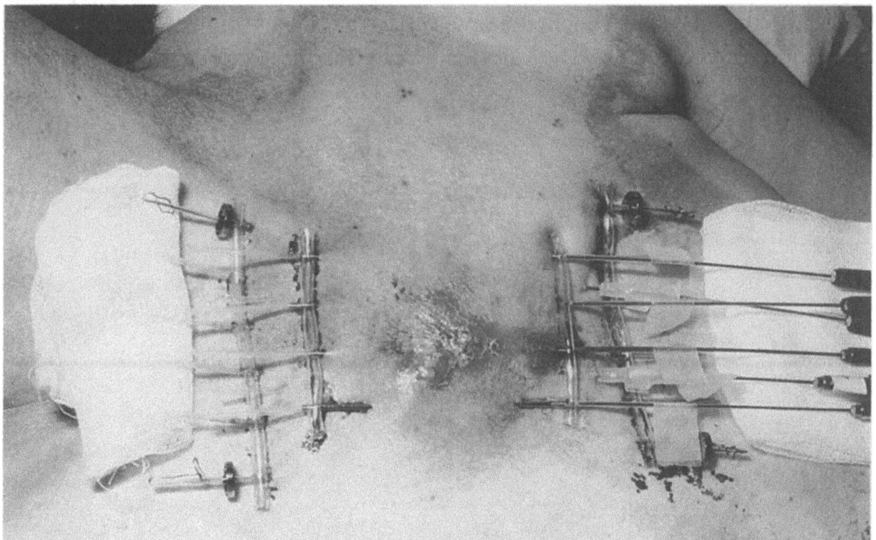

Fig. 1.10. Biplanar implantation for a large chest wall relapse of a breast cancer. RF technique with the Villejuif metal–plastic tubes

tion is chest wall relapse of breast cancer, the deep implantation being limited by the ribs. In such cases two solutions can be considered: Firstly a row of electrodes may be implanted as deep as possible. The use of this row would lead to an "underheating" of the superficial millimeters. These superficial layers can be heated by a complementary external system; since only 2 or 3 mm need additional heating, we can use here, for example, cushions filled with hot water or simple infrared lamps [51, 73]. Accurate measurement of temperature at as many points as possible is mandatory [30]. The second and preferable solution consists in the placement of a second superficial row of needles or tubes, just in contact or 1–3 mm above the skin (or the tumor). This type of application is made possible by the external immobilization template systems described above. To obtain electrical contact between the metallic portions of the probes and the underlying skin (or tumor), we must fill the free space under the electrodes with a conductive jelly (such as ECG jelly). Again, accurate thermometry is mandatory, since large differences between the conductivities of the jelly and of the tumor can lead to severe burns. Actually, it is particularly easy to insert several thermocouples or thermistors in the jelly to make sure there are not hot spots at the skin (tumor)-jelly interface. If such hot spots are observed, we have to look for another type of jelly whose electrical conductivity is lower (such as the classical ultrasound one). Since the brachytherapists are used to performing "plesiotherapy" [radioactive material at point of contact with the tumor, or with a few millimeters free space (air) between the radioactive wires or seeds and the tumor], such a type of application is perfectly suitable for them. Such an implantation is shown in Fig. 1.11.

When working with the *microwave radiative technique*, the implantation procedure is much easier. In this case the classical brachytherapy tubes are implanted exactly in the way they are for brachytherapy (see previous description of the implantation of the low frequency hyperthermia tubes and [101]). Some rules must, however, be obeyed.

The *number of probes* depends on the size of the tumor and on the possible spacing of the microwave antennae. We previously saw (Sect. 1.2.5.3) that, at least theoretically, the spacing of the microwave probes could be a little larger than the spacing which is required for low frequency electrodes. Hence some authors implant their tubes 2 cm apart. Others consider this spacing suitable for hyperthermia, but incorrect for brachytherapy. Consequently they implant their plastic tubes every centimeter. They insert the microwave antennae 2 cm apart using the intermediate row of tubes solely for thermometry. For brachytherapy, all the tubes are loaded with iridium 192 seeds or wires. Anyway, as previously stated, a 2 cm spacing is not always optimal with microwaves and it seems advisable to implant the tubes with a spacing of about 1.5 cm.

The *length of the heating part* along a given line is not related in this case to the implanted material, but to the type of antenna which will be inserted in it. When implanting the plastic tubes, the clinician must take into account the maximum length he is able to heat with his available material. When a large tumor has to be treated and when the antennae can only heat a 5 cm length, for example, a solution can be to divide the volume into two segments lengthwise and heat each half separately. Another solution could be the insertion of two antennae by each exteriorized end of the plastic tubes. These solutions are not really satisfactory and more sophisticated antennae [123] or development of the modified 27 MHz technique [83] are eagerly awaited.

The *number of planes* is not a problem with microwaves: a monoplanar implant of antennae can heat a slightly thicker volume than the radiofrequency technique. Since every antenna can act independently, any

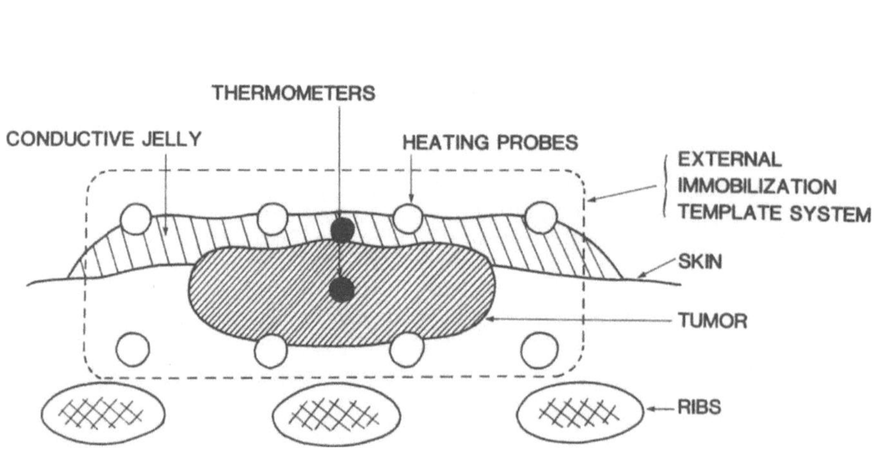

Fig. 1.11. RF technique: "plesiotherapy" application. Electrical contact by conductive jelly

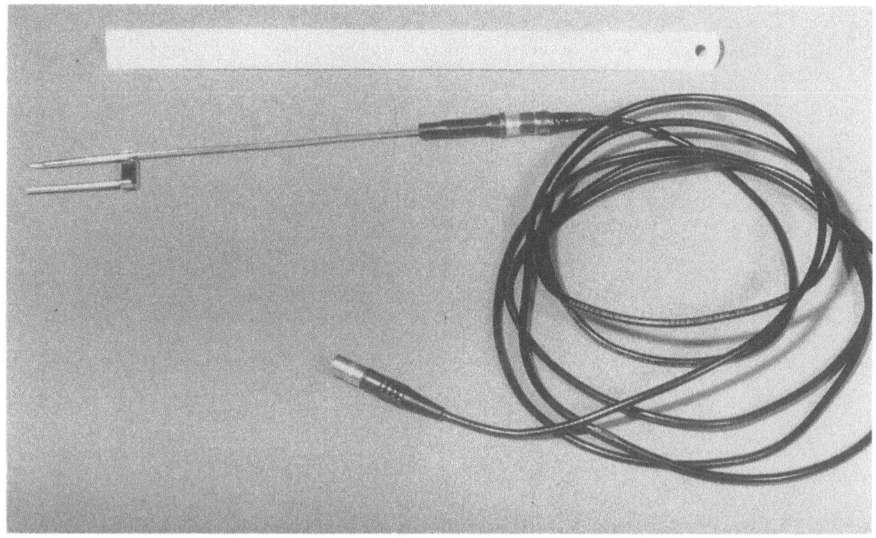

Fig. 1.12. Direct connecting of the RF probe to the metallic hairpin guide used for brachytherapy implantation of cancers of the tongue. (Courtesy of J. C. Horiot and P. Janoray, Dijon, France)

number of rows can be used without any limitation. The requirements concerning the *geometry* are approximately the same as for the previous technique: any lack of parallelism leads to hot or cold spots. The immobilization of the implanted system can be achieved with the procedures described above.

1.3.1.3 Techniques of Implantation for Head and Neck Primary Tumors

We shall not consider further the techniques for the implantation of *neck nodes*. From a technical point of view these lesions can be equated with superficial tumors, and the clinician usually selects one of the procedures described in the previous section.
The different types of implantation which are possible for head and neck *primary tumors* will be discussed. Most patients who have been treated so far by the interstitial hyperthermia-brachytherapy combination for head and neck lesions presented with tumors of the tongue (base and/or anterior two-thirds) or of the floor of the mouth.
With the exception of a technique used in Dijon (which will be described below) all the implant techniques for primary head and neck tumors require a general anesthetic.
For *radiofrequency resistive diathermy*, several types of implanted material can be considered, all the procedures aiming at obtaining the classical "loop" necessary for the subsequent brachytherapy application. The group at Villejuif, France, began with an adaptation of the "metal-plastic" tubes, designing special tubes for head and neck tumors. These hyperthermia tubes consisted of two metallic parts to be implanted in parallel, and of a plastic intermediate "bridge." The two metallic parts were connected to the generator, forming a classical pair of electrodes of the radiofrequency technique. The tubes were subsequently loaded with iridium 192 wires according to the usual brachytherapy technique. Utilized only for a few patients, this technique had the advantage of specifically heating the tumor, and of completely sparing the skin and the subcutaneous healthy tissues. In addition, if necessary, a second hyperthermia session could be performed after the brachytherapy period.
However, this sophisticated technique was found to present several drawbacks. The implantation of such "multipart" tubes was rather difficult. In addition there was a serious problem of disconnection of the different parts during the insertion and removal of the tubes. This technique was therefore abandoned.
At Stanford, about a dozen patients have been treated utilizing the special hyperthermia tubes (plastic tubes coated with a thin metal layer). No technical problem has been reported to date.
At Dijon, France, a technique was developed taking advantage of the metallic hairpin guides which are implanted in the tongue prior to the insertion of hairpin iridium 192 wires [35, 101]. The hairpin guides are directly connected to the low frequency generator by inserting the coaxial probe of the amplifier into one of the two "legs" of the guides (see Fig. 1.12). In this technique the hyperthermia session is given immediately, then the hairpin iridium wire is inserted in the guide, and this guide removed. This means that only one hyperthermia session can be given prior to brachytherapy. Using this technique, one problem emerged: burns were observed in some cases just under the "bridge" binding the two legs of the hairpin

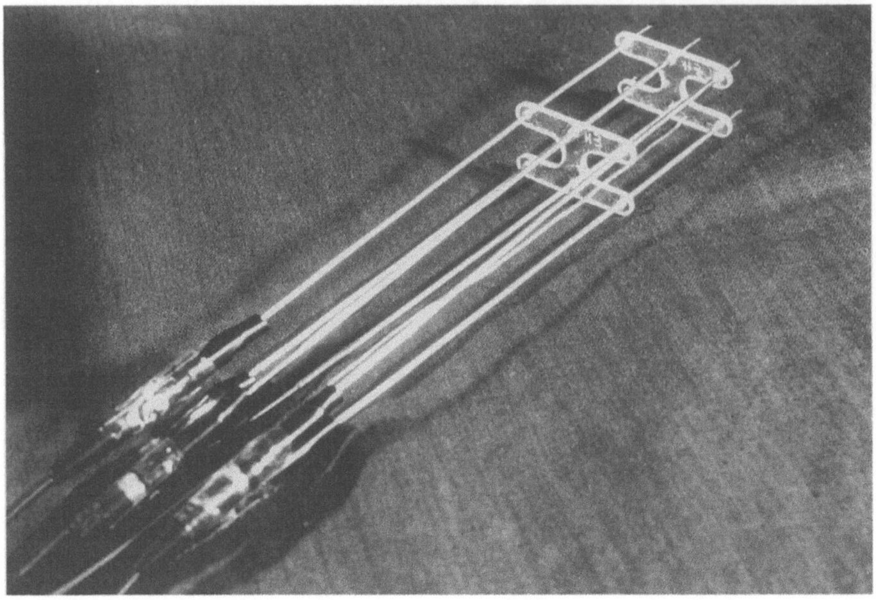

Fig. 1.13. Template immobilization system for an implantation of a tongue cancer. RF technique. (Courtesy of J.P. Gerard and G. De Laroche, Lyon, France)

guide. To prevent this complication, the Dijon group is now considering the use of special hairpin guides whose bridge is made of a nonconductive material (such as plastic). With these new guides, it will be necessary to connect each leg of the hairpin to the generator.

A modified method is now used in several centers. The implantation begins as a classical brachytherapy one, with the insertion of parallel metallic needles. Once all the needles are implanted according to the desired geometry, they can be connected to the low frequency amplifier. Some kind of insulation (varnish, or more commonly plastic catheters overcoating the proximal parts of the needles) prevents any heating of the skin and of the subcutaneous tissue, except if the tumor involves these structures. Plastic templates can be used to achieve good parallel geometry with the needles (Fig. 1.13). The tip of the needles in the mouth can occasionally make contact with the palate, resulting in local but sometimes severe palatal burns. This complication can be simply prevented by the use of an insulation material (e.g., plastic plate or rubber sheet) which is placed between the tip of the needles and the palate.

Once the hyperthermia session is completed, the clinician can proceed with the usual brachytherapy technique: insertion of nylon guides through the needles, removal of the needles, placement of the plastic tubes by overcoating of the nylon guides (see Fig. 1.6), and finally loading of the tubes by iridium 192 wires or seeds.

This technique has the main advantage that it fits in well with the successive steps of a typical brachytherapy implant, only delaying the insertion of the plastic tubes for about 45 min. Obviously, only one hyperthermia session can be performed prior to brachytherapy, as for the Dijon technique, but this is not a drawback for the groups whose treatment schedules plan only one prebrachytherapy interstitial hyperthermia session. The details of this technique are shown in Fig. 1.14.

The rules for the total number of probes, the number of rows, the length of the heating parts, and the geometry can be easily extrapolated from what has been defined in Sect. 1.3.1.2 (superficial lesions). When considering the spacing of the probes, we must mention a clinical problem which arose at Villejuif and at Stanford (G. Hahn, personal communication). For some base of tongue tumors, a "classical" spacing of 1.2–1.5 cm led to important temperature gradients. In one Villejuif patient it was impossible to obtain more than 42 °C in the center of a square cross-sectional area of a volume encompassed by four needles spaced 1.5 cm apart and heated at 45 °C. For this patient it was necessary to use the "central" metallic needle (initially implanted for the sole use of thermometry) as a heating probe: it was then possible to achieve a temperature of 44 °C in all electrodes, in spite of the odd number.

These surprisingly large temperature inhomogeneities which were observed in spite of "good" implant geometry could possibly be related to a high perfusion rate of some base of tongue tumors.

When working with the *microwave antennae*, the problem is once again simpler. The classical plastic tube implant performed for brachytherapy is perfectly

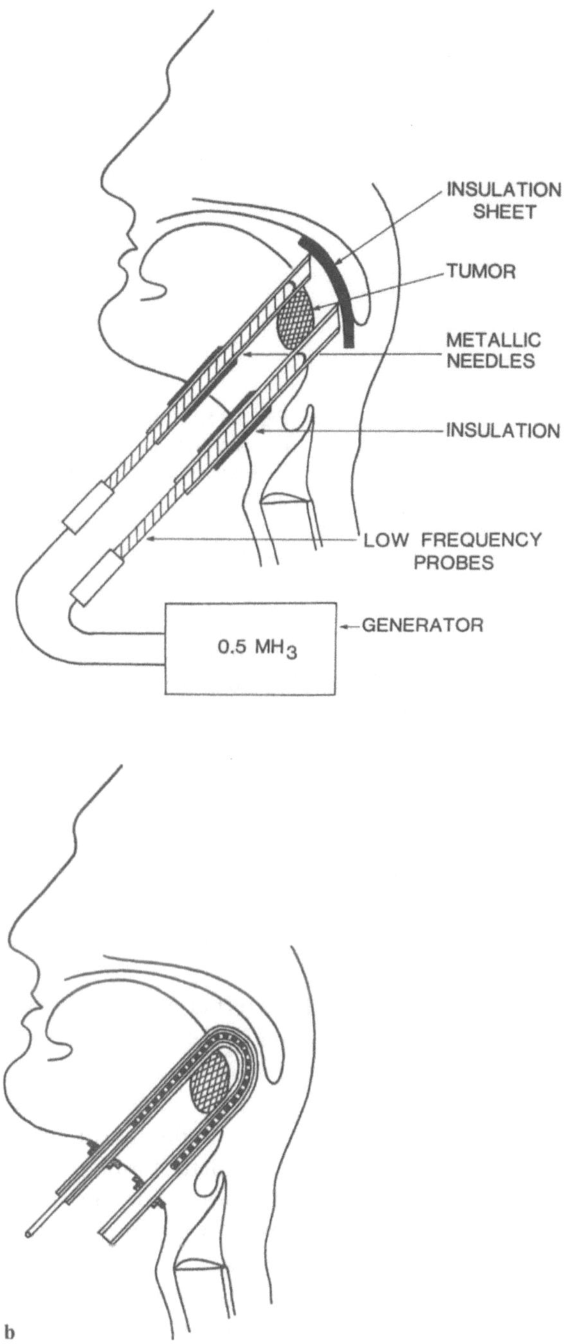

Fig. 1.14a, b. RF technique: implantation for a cancer of the base of the tongue. **a** Hyperthermia technique. **b** Brachytherapy: placement of the classical plastic tubes and loading with iridium 192 seeds or wires

suitable for microwave radiative heating. The spacing of the tubes should be in the range 1.5–2 cm (1.5 cm advisable). When loading the loops, the classical 915 MHz antennae are usually too short to make possible a correct heating of the volume to be treated. In this case, *two* antennae must be inserted, in each exteriorized end of the same plastic tube. This problem will be overcome if longer antennae become available.

1.3.1.4 Techniques of Implantation for Pelvic Tumors

When working with microwave antennae, is should be theoretically possible to take advantage of the plastic tube implants performed for bladder or prostate cancers in some centers [101]. However, most of the implantations which have been performed so far for pelvic tumors have utilized metallic needles connected to a low frequency amplifier. It is not advisable to insert microwave antennae in such metallic needles: the high temperature which would be achieved at the surface of the needle would lead to a high risk of burns. We will therefore focus on the radiofrequency technique. All these sophisticated applications require some type of template. These applicators have two roles: firstly they are a major parameter of the geometric quality of the application (parallelism); secondly, they ensure that the spacing between the probes is and remains the same (at least for the distal – external – parts of the needles) during the whole brachytherapy application. For pelvic interstitial hyperthermia, we actually use the templates which have been designed for brachytherapy implants. Usually these immobilization devices are designed for a specific tumor site: the Syed-Neblett "butterfly" for parametrial implantations [57], the vaginal template used at Lyon, France, for centropelvic tumors and relapses located at the distal part of the vagina, the Syed-Neblett rectal template [129] most similar to the device developed by the Lyon group [37], the Syed-Neblett prostate template [130], and others [4]. On the other hand, Martinez et al. [85, 86] developed an original multiple-site single applicator which can also be used for interstitial hyperthermia implants.

All these implantations are obviously performed with the patient under general anesthesia. Two types of needle can be used: the classical metallic needles which are currently utilized in the first step of the usual brachytherapy implantations (see previous sections), or the special needles designed by Syed [106, 132]. The latter consist of two parts: an "external" hollow needle whose tip is rounded, and an "internal" piece whose tip is sharp pointed. To insert the material, the internal piece is pushed into the hollow needle until the sharp tip shows out of the round tip of the external piece. The sharp extremity allows the clinician to easily implant the material through the skin. Once the skin has been passed through, the internal sharp guide is removed and the round-tip needle is

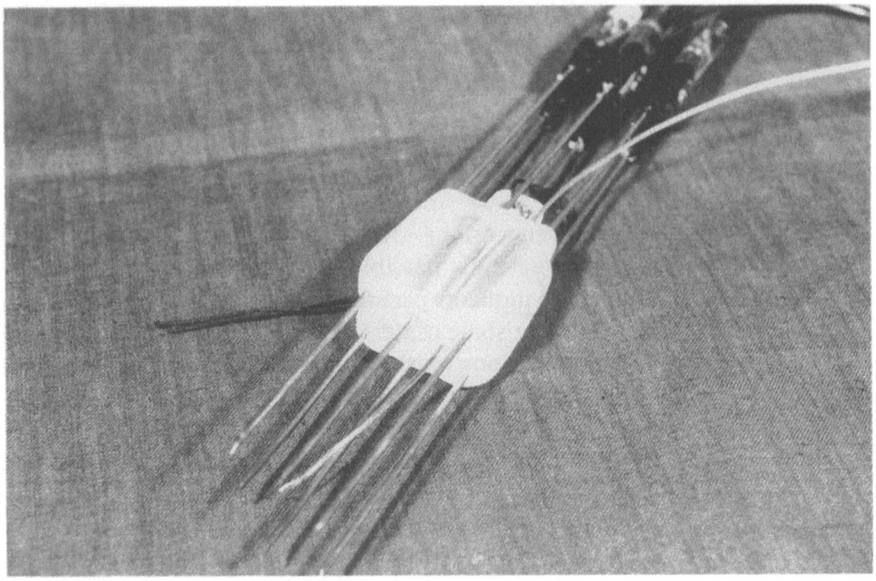

Fig. 1.15. Template immobilization system for a localized recurrence of a corpus uteri cancer. RF technique. (Courtesy of J.P. Gerard and G. De Laroche, Lyon, France)

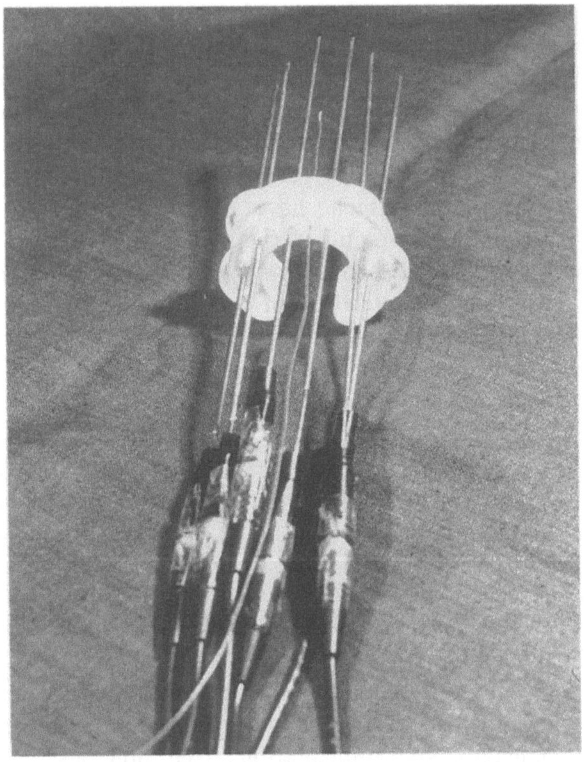

Fig. 1.16. Template immobilization system for an implantation for a rectal cancer. RF technique. (Courtesy of J.P. Gerard and G. De Laroche, Lyon, Paris)

gently pushed until it is in a suitable position. This technique has been developed in order to avoid transfixion of normal structures such as arteries or small bowel.

The number of needles to be implanted depends on the site and on the size of the tumor to be treated. In some unusual situations, four to six needles are enough to encompass the tumor volume (see Fig. 1.15). For rectal cancers, six to ten needles are usually required (see. Figs. 1.16, 1.17). For a large bilateral parametrial implantations – for example for a cancer of the uterine cervix stage III –, up to 40 needles may be necessary (see Fig. 1.18).

The spacing should be in the usual range, e.g., 1.2–1.5 cm.

While the parallelism of the external parts of the implanted needles is always good (these parts are firmly maintained by the immobilization template), this is not always the case for the "internal" ends of the needles in the pelvis. When long needles have to be implanted (essentially for parametrial tumoral involvement), they can slightly diverge and we sometimes have to accept a geometry of the implantation which is not entirely satisfactory.

More and more groups throughout the world are presently involved in pelvic implantations for brachytherapy, possibly combined with hyperthermia [4, 105, 139].

1.3.2 Heating Technique

The way the low frequency amplifier is connected to the implanted material is of paramount importance in the resistive technique. Any error in the connections would lead to an inability to achieve a satisfactory distribution of temperature. Each pair of probes must therefore be carefully and clearly identified.

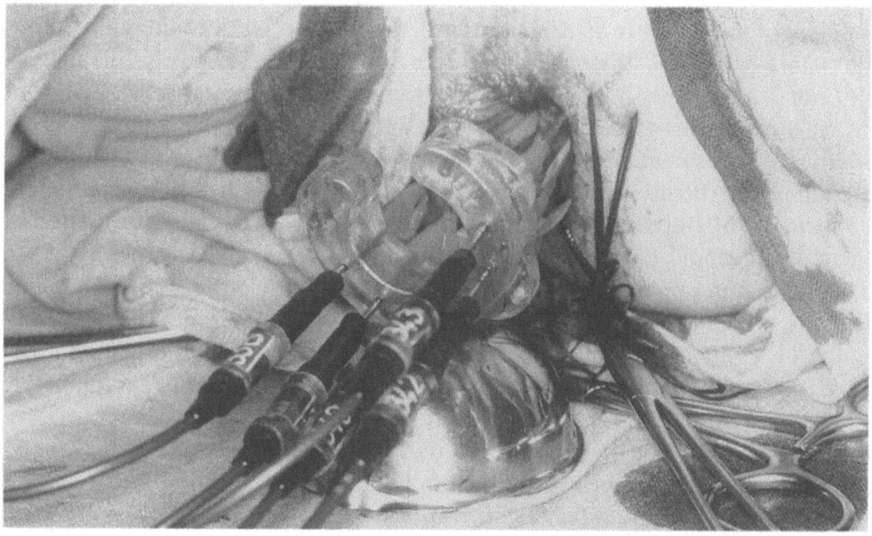

Fig. 1.17. Implantation for interstitial RF thermoradiotherapy of a rectal cancer. (Courtesy of J. P. Gerard and G. De Laroche, Lyon, France)

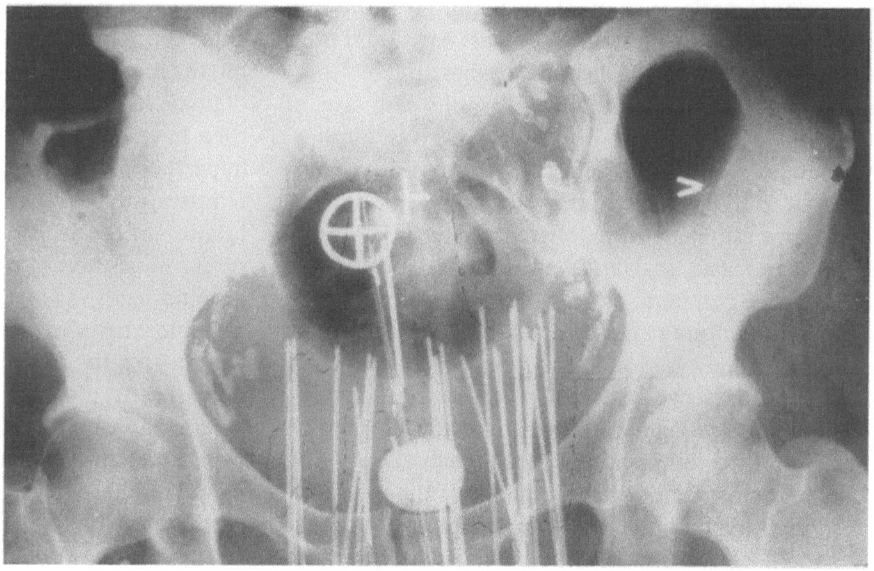

Fig. 1.18. Multineedle pelvic implantation for a relapse of a cancer of the uterine cervix. RF technique

On the other hand, since the microwave antennae are radiating independently, the insertion of this material in the plastic tubes does not pose a problem.
During the hyperthermia sessions, we have to face two very different situations: when the patient is awake (with or without a light sedation), and when the patient is under general anesthesia. These situations will now be considered.

1.3.2.1 Patients Awake, With or Without Sedation

In this case we have to keep in mind that a rapid (e.g., 30 s) increase in the temperature, even if it only reaches a moderate level (41 °– 42 °C), is not well tolerated by patients. However, this same rise can be tolerated if it takes place over 3 – 5 min.
According to our clinical experience, we would first recommend having the patient under light sedation. Secondly we usually progressively increase the power in the probes in successive steps in order to achieve 40 °C in all heating electrodes, then 42 °C, then 44 °C, and possibly more if it proves necessary to achieve the usually prescribed minimum temperature of 44 °C at the center of the application. Most of the time, it takes 8 – 10 min to achieve this goal, and sometimes more. If it is too high, the temperature in the heating lines can pose a problem. The usual pain threshold that we observed in our patients (without any sedation) was 45 °C. This threshold can usually be slightly

increased (to 45.5 °–46 °C) with light sedation. This biological "red light" is of clinical use: if the patient complains while all the measured points indicate 44 °C or less, it usually means that the temperature has reached at least 45 °C somewhere in a small area. Additional measurements, all along the plastic tubes implanted for the use of thermometry, usually allow the location of this area (often an old scar).

The pain threshold may vary somewhat from patient to patient, but is extremely "sharp" for a given patient. A patient who complains at 45 °C usually stands 44 °C after a minimal reduction of the applied power.

We shall see later that a usual thermal dose prescription is 43 °–44 °C for 45–60 min. To date most authors agree that the temperature which must be taken into account is the *minimum* temperature measured within the heated volume. Thus the regulation of the power (automatic or manual, depending on the machine) should aim at obtaining at least 43 °C and preferably 44 °C not in the heating probes, but in some additional catheters implanted for the sole use of thermometry, usually at the center of a given implication, as far as possible from the heating lines (where the SAR is likely to be lower, except if working with microwave antennae in a coherent system) [31, 55].

In the best cases, an almost uniform distribution of temperature can be obtained, the same (or about the same) temperature being achieved both in the heating lines and in the additional catheters. Often we recorded slight difference between heating electrodes and thermometry catheters, in the range 0.5 °–1 °C. This means that the temperature should reach about 45 °C (thus very close to the pain threshold) if the minimum prescribed temperature is 44 °C (the results obtained in patient series will be reported in detail in Sect. 1.3.5).

Once a satisfactory temperature distribution is achieved, a *constant* applied power permits a plateau temperature to be maintained during the prescribed 45 min in about half of the cases. In the order half, we have observed a general temperature *increase* in all the probes, while the power remained *constant* after 35–40 min of hyperthermia at 44 °C (minimum temperature). This could be interpreted as a decrease in blood flow, due to capillary collapse and blood stasis. Considering the large amount of data recently reported by Reinhold in his extensive review, it seems quite possible that our thermal dose of 44 °C for 45 min is approximately the threshold dose for microcirculation collapse [108]. This could explain why this phenomenon has not been observed in all our patients. The possible factors involved in this blood flow decrease are numerous: recently no less than 11 successive parameters possibly involved in this hyperthermia-induced circulatory dysfunction were listed [108].

Clinically this means that in a significant number of cases we observe a rapid temperature rise at the end of the hyperthermia session. The problem can be easily overcome by the immediate reduction of the applied power either manually or automatically (in the machines regulated by feedback from a given thermometric probe).

At least for the manually operated machines, this underlines the need for some type of safety device to prevent the temperature from exceeding a certain value (usually the pain threshold, about 45 °–46 °C) in *all* the heating lines.

1.3.2.2 Patients Under General Anesthesia

This way of heating is obviously much more comfortable for the patient, and also for the clinician operating the machine. In such cases the desired temperature plateau can be achieved much faster, in 2–3 min. We then have to face a new problem: after 7–10 min of hyperthermia, the applied power being constant, the temperature falls off, due to heat-induced vascular dilatation of the arterioles as well as the veins [108]. The power must therefore be *increased*, either manually or automatically. (This phenomenon is generally indiscernible when the patient is awake, because it then occurs *during* the period of the regulation of the power necessary to increase slowly the probe temperatures.)

At the end of the hyperthermia application, a *reduction* of the applied power may be necessary in a significant number of cases, as described in the previous section.

1.3.3 Brachytherapy Technique

The technique of brachytherapy to be used in conjunction with interstitial hyperthermia is similar to the "classical" one.

We previously saw that an afterloading technique should be used. The radioactive material which is usually employed is iridium 192 (wires in Europe, seeds in North America).

The choice of the activity of the iridium wires or seeds deserves further discussion. At the beginning of the hyperthermia era, the radiosensitizing effect was emphasized while direct heat toxicity was considered to be of less clinical value. When working with interstitial hyperthermia in combination with a low dose rate irradiation, it was felt that the brachytherapy period should take place as close as possible to the hyperthermia and in the shortest time possible (the radiosensitizing effect of hyperthermia being lost in a few hours). Thus in several treatment schedules, brachytherapy started immediately after hyperthermia and the usual 40 Gy was given in, for example, 2 days. This is shorter than the usual brachytherapy duration time, most groups, at least in Europe, delivering only 10 Gy per day. With better understanding of the fundamental mechanisms of hyperthermia and with increasing clinical experience, this prescription of a "short time" brachytherapy (thus with a high iridium 192 activity) may be discussed. The sensitizing effect achieved just after the hyperthermia session could be detrimental for normal tissues included in the treatment volume. Moreover, this effect is completely lost after 4–6 h: thus hyperthermia sensitizes only a small part of the brachytherapy irradiation, during the first few hours. It would be unlikely to achieve a significant increase in the biological effect by only sensitizing the first 5–6 Gy! Nevertheless, the TER of such an association was estimated to be in the order of 2, and perhaps more, by Manning, according to his clinical experience [82]. From the clinical experience in Villejuif [34] and from experimental data from Dijon, France [70], this TER was felt to be in the range of 1.5–2. This indicates that radiosensitization may not be the only factor involved. In fact, at the present time, for the "external" associations of irradiation and heat it is felt that direct heat cytotoxicity is the most important parameter, focusing on hypoxic and nutritionally deprived cells (the ones most likely to be radioresistant), the radiosensitization playing only a small part.

In conclusion, the interstitial hyperthermia–brachytherapy combination may be effective more as a "spatial" complementary effect (with different cell targets) than because of radiosensitization.

Clinically, this means that the duration of brachytherapy could be less critical than was recently tought: all "classical" schedules could be accepted (for example from 10 to 25 Gy per day). Although it has still to be unequivocally proven in clinical practice, it is unlikely that different brachytherapy durations produce very different clinical results.

During the brachytherapy period the problems which can arise are exactly the same as are experienced with classical brachytherapy applications. Additional medical treatment (sedatives, steroids, antibiotics) may be necessary [101].

The superficial implantations are usually well tolerated. The head and neck implantations are less comfortable, but light sedation and steroids usually make the applications tolerable.. In our experience, the pelvic implants (essentially the large multineedle parametrial implantations) are poorly tolerated and need strong analgesics (usually regular opiates).

The radioactive wires or seeds can be removed at any time and anywhere. On the other hand, the removal of the implanted needles or tubes must be performed with great care: electively in the operating room, with an anesthesist present.

The possible overheating around the implanted probes combined with the small volume of "overdose" around the iridium seeds or wires leads in almost all cases to a small channel of necrosis all around the probes. When removing this material, bleeding can occur. Simple compression is usually enough, but the clinician must be prepared for possible surgical intervention if required.

Another potential problem can occur when removing the three-part metallic–plastic tubes: the component parts can disconnect at the time of removal. It is thus strongly advised to insert a guide (usually a nylon wire) in the tube, keeping the two ends of the guide exteriorized when removing the three-part tube. In case of disconnection, a part of the tube remaining in the tumor can be pushed out using an ordinary plastic tube overcoating the nylon guide.

It should also be known that the regression of the tumor after hyperthermia–brachytherapy is usually faster than is observed after brachytherapy alone (due to the "immediate" cell toxicity of hyperthermia and/or vascular damage). Hence complete or partial responses are frequently observed at the time of removal of the implantation material.

This has been observed in the Villejuif experience [33]. Linares, at the Memorial Cancer Center of New York, also noted a striking initial response in some patients, with tumor liquefaction and marked tumor necrosis, so that an almost 50% reduction in tumor volume occurred within the first few days after the hyperthermia session [78].

1.3.4 Treatment Schedule

Just as with external hyperthermia, it is widely agreed that interstitial hyperthermia should be used in combination with radiation. In all studies, hyperthermia *alone* has been shown to yield poor results [14]. Even when a good or complete response was achieved, rapid local relapse was an almost universal finding [29]. Unfortunately, the practical details of the optimal way of combining interstitial hyperthermia and irradiation have not yet been settled. The reason for this is probably that not enough biological data on the association of interstitial hyperthermia and low dose rate irradiation have been available to allow the clinicians to define the best treatment schedule. In addition there have been practical clinical limitations: it is generally agreed that the duration of a hyperthermia session cannot exceed approximately 1 h, either because of patient discomfort (if awake) or because extended periods of general anesthesia are unacceptable.

The treatment protocols which have been used so far in different centers will be reviewed, and the design of future protocols considered.

Only one author in the literature (Yabumoto et al. [143]) combined a technique of interstitial hyperthermia with external beam radiotherapy (in a short series of seven patients). All the other groups used a combination of interstitial hyperthermia and brachytherapy, or added to this combination a (moderate) dose of external beam irradiation.

The group at the University of Arizona, Tuscon [80, 82, 94], proposed a simple combination of interstitial hyperthermia and brachytherapy. Hyperthermia was given first, a temperature of 42.5 °–43 °C being delivered for 30 min.. The loading of the implanted material took place 1–2 h after the hyperthermia session was completed. A wide range of radiation doses was given in the 17 patients reported in the first paper [82]. Nine patients were given a dose of 20–30 Gy, and eight a dose of 40–45 Gy. No second hyperthermia session was given after brachytherapy. The clinical results will be discussed in a following section.

Joseph et al., at the City of Hope National Medical Center, reported on seven patients in an early paper (1981) [72]. The proposed schedule combined external beam radiotherapy (30–40 Gy in 3–4 weeks), and, after a 3-week rest, a first session of interstitial hyperthermia (41 °–43 °C for 30 min), then brachytherapy (20–30 Gy), and finally a second interstitial hyperthermia session (41 °–43 °C for 30 min).

In a subsequent paper from the same group, Vora et al. [138] reported 16 implanted lesions in 15 patients with relatively large variations of the protocol from one case to another. In previously untreated patients, the external radiation treatment was in the range of 45–50 Gy and the interstitial implant dose in the range of 15–30 Gy. In this second series, interstitial hyperthermia was only given prior to interstitial irradiation, except in selected cases where the radiation dose was reduced due to prior treatment, and for which a second hyperthermia treatment was given after brachytherapy.

At the Institut Gustave-Roussy, Villejuif, France, the first protocol which was developed in 1981 was an adaptation of that used in Tucson [31]. It only combined interstitial hyperthermia and brachytherapy. Hyperthermia was given first and the minimum target temperature was 44 °C in the selected volume for 45 min. Immediately after hyperthermia was completed, the tubes were loaded with iridium 192 wires. A dose of 30 Gy was given to the first 17 patients. After two local relapses were observed in this early series, the dose was increased to 40 Gy for the following applications [34].

Bicher et al. [13], in Inglewood, California, proposed a very sophisticated protocol combining external irradiation, interstitial hyperthermia, and brachytherapy. A first interstitial irradiation (25 Gy) was given in week 1, with interstitial hyperthermia (42 °–45 °C for 1 h) before and after brachytherapy. In week 2, four fractions of 2 Gy (external radiotherapy) were delivered. In week 3, a new series of interstitial thermoradiotherapy sessions was given, similar to that given in week 1. Hence the total irradiation dose was 50 Gy (interstitial) + 8 Gy (external), combined with four hyperthermia sessions (42 °–45 °C for 1 h).

Puthawala and Syed from Long Beach (California) recently reported on 44 patients receiving interstitial thermoradiotherapy for salvage of recurrent and/or persistent squamous cell carcinoma of the head and neck [107]. An interstitial irradiation was given at doses of 40–60 Gy over a period of 80–120 h (i.e., a dose rate of about 0.50 Gy/h), with two interstitial heat applications, before and after brachytherapy, delivering 42 °–43 °C for 60 min on each occasion. For recurrent malignant tumors from other sites, they used the same type of treatment schedule [106, 132].

The group from St. Louis, Missouri (Emami et al. [55]), recently updated their results and reported 48 recurrent/persistent tumors treated in 46 patients. For their interstitial hyperthermia applications they specified a minimum tumor temperature of 42.5 °–43 °C for 60 min. Nine patients were treated by a combination of interstitial hyperthermia and external beam radiation therapy. The total irradiation dose was 30–40 Gy. Four to six hyperthermia sessions were given. Nine other patients received only interstitial thermoradiotherapy, but with only one session of hyperthermia prior to irradiation. Most of the patients (30) received a protocol combining *brachytherapy* and two interstitial hyperthermia sessions, before and after irradiation. While the heat applications, as described above, were relatively homogeneous, the irradiation doses varied over a wide range, from 20 to 60 Gy (delivered in 4–7 days), depending on the previous radiation dosage received by the patient.

In his series of ten patients, Linares [78], at the Memorial Cancer Center in New York, interstitially heated the patients for 45 min at the plateau with a control sensor set at 43.5 °C (minimum temperature?). One session was given for five patients, and two for the other five. This author combined interstitial hyperthermia either with external or interstitial irradiation, or both.

All these data are somewhat confusing: The hyperthermia sessions varied from center to center (temperature level, duration) and even in a given center. (What is the meaning of "42°–45°C" for 1 h? The antitumor efficacy of 42°C for 1 h is obviously not the same as that of 45°C for 1 h.) There was also a wide variety of radiation doses, and of sequencing of the interstitial hyperthermia–radiation combination. The following questions should be considered:

1. What temperature should be accepted as the "treatment temperature" for a given study?
2. What is the optimal duration of an interstitial heat application?
3. What is the optimal number of interstitial hyperthermia sessions?
4. Should we use external and/or interstitial irradiation?
5. Which radiation dose should be given?
6. What is the best method of sequencing combinations of hyperthermia and radiation?

1.3.4.1 What Temperature Should Be Accepted as the "Treatment Temperature"?

The data reviewed in the above section show that the therapeutic temperature was sometimes not precisely defined; it is important to know if it corresponds to the minimum, the maximum, or the "mean" temperature.

It appears dangerous to rely on the maximum, or even the "mean" temperature achieved in the treated volume. This way of presenting the data may overlook cold spots in the treatment volume, with consequent suboptimal tumor cell killing.

There is now general agreement that the *minimum* estimated temperature which was achieved in the tumor volume should be used to describe the treatment. The other measurement points can be taken into account to assess the homogeneity (i.e., the quality of the temperature distribution) but they must *not* be considered for the "protocol definition" of thermal dose. We shall see in Sect. 1.3.6 that the minimum temperature has been shown to correlate with complete response rate in domestic animals [44] and in man [3, 32, 55, 94]. It is thus the accepted temperature to consider in protocol definition.

1.3.4.2 What Is the Optimal Duration of an Interstitial Heat Application?

From a practical point of view, the hyperthermia session cannot exceed approximately 1 h. Most authors propose a duration in the range of 40–60 min for each hyperthermia session. The minimum temperature should, of course, be the highest possible. We would therefore advise 43.5°–44°C for 45–60 min, being aware of the fact that in some instances it will be impossible to reach this level. In those cases, additional interstitial hyperthermia sessions should be considered.

1.3.4.3 What Is the Optimal Number of Interstitial Hyperthermia Sessions?

The optimal number of interstitial hyperthermia sessions clearly depends on their quality. It appears that only one session of interstitial hyperthermia, reaching a minimum temperature of 44°C for 45 min, and given prior to the interstitial irradiation, is highly effective [34, 82]. This scheme presents several advantages: it is simple (only one hyperthermia application); it avoids all the problems of thermotolerance which are likely to occur if a second session is given within a short time after the first one; and it fits well with the implantation techniques performed during a single general anesthetic prior to brachytherapy (see Sect. 1.3.1).

It remains that, in a significant proportion of cases, a minimum temperature of 44°C cannot be achieved. In these cases, a second hyperthermia session is advisable. A minimum temperature of 43°C can often be achieved with the generators presently available. We can expect that the efficacy of two sessions for 43°C for 60 min will be similar to one fraction of 44°C for 60 min (in the absence of thermotolerance).

It is worth observing that the complete response rates reported clinically with 44°C for 45 min and brachytherapy are close to those noted after the schedule 43°C–60 min, brachytherapy, 43°C–60 min (see Sect. 1.3.6).

1.3.4.4 External and/or Interstitial Irradiation?

The mixture of external and interstitial irradiation in some papers makes the evaluation of technique rather difficult. In fact, the schedule "external radiotherapy and interstitial thermoradiotherapy" has often been proposed for those patients who have not previously

received any radiotherapy, as a tentative improvement on the traditional combination of external radiotherapy and brachytherapy (e.g., for cancers of the tongue or uterine cervix).
On the other hand, interstitial thermoradiotherapy alone has so far been essentially proposed for relapses in *previously irradiated* areas, in the hope that hyperthermia combined with low dose rate irradiation could be well tolerated by the previously treated healthy tissues.

1.3.4.5 Which Radiation Dose Should Be Given?

The range of radiation doses which have been given so far by different authors is striking; it varies from 20 to 60 Gy. However, on closer analysis of the data the reasons for this apparent discrepancy can be more readily understood.
When patients had been previously heavily irradiated, it is understandable that the clinicians were reluctant to retreat with high radiation doses. In those cases, they usually limited their doses to 20–30 Gy.
When patients had received accepted radical radiotherapy courses of radiation (such as postoperative radiotherapy for breast cancer to doses of 45–50 Gy), most clinicians tried to deliver a dose of 30–50 Gy (brachytherapy) combined with hyperthermia.
In patients who had not had prior radiotherapy, it could be expected that hyperthermia would increase the local control rate without adding much toxicity (this will be further discussed in Sect. 1.4.4). In these circumstances, clinicians usually kept the traditional radiation dose (or sometimes slightly decreased it) – 60 Gy.
For the future, it will certainly be useful to design separate and precise protocols for relapses in previously irradiated volumes and for tumors which have not received any prior treatment.

1.3.4.6 What Is the Best Sequence?

A few biological data are available concerning the combination of hyperthermia with low dose rate irradiation [9, 10, 90, 116], but no data are available so far showing that heat should be administered before or after brachytherapy.
As previously emphasized in Sect. 1.3.3, the sensitization of irradiation by hyperthermia is probably a minor phenomenon in this interstitial thermoradiotherapy combination. The results are more likely to be explained by an additional and complementary effect of the two treatment modalities. If this hypothesis is correct, the chronology is perhaps of minor importance.
On the other hand, it is much more comfortable for the patient and the clinician to have the hyperthermia performed during general anesthesia which is usually mandatory for the implantation of the afterloading material, and thus *before* the brachytherapy treatment period.
Finally, even if we cannot presently define the optimal protocols, we can at least try to draw up some guidelines.
It seems clear that we have to consider separately patients not previously treated and the relapses in irradiated areas. For patients not previously treated it seems advisable to keep the "classical" radiation dose and simply to add interstitial hyperthermia (this is in agreement with the guiding principles of the three first clinical trials – for external hyperthermia – designed by the European Society for Hyperthermic Oncology [97]. The radiotherapy can be either brachytherapy alone or a combination of external irradiation and brachytherapy.
For patients presenting with relapses in previously irradiated areas, the irradiation dose has to be reduced. Some biological data (Janoray et al. [70]) suggest that 44 °C for 45 min and 40 Gy brachytherapy could be as efficient as 65–70 Gy with less toxicity in some situations. Three French centers working together accepted such a protocol, i.e., 43.5 °–44 °C (minimum temperature) and 40 Gy [37]. However, as emphasized by Emami [55], if the previous treatment already delivered a large dose of radiation, the dose must be reduced to 20–30 Gy.

1.3.5 Distribution of Temperatures in Patients

As we shall see in the next section, the distribution of the temperature throughout the tumor volume, as would be expected, is one of the parameters which governs the tumor response.
Unfortunately, this precise distribution has not been systematically reported in the papers published so far, probably partly because the optimal way to report these technical results has not yet been settled.
Joseph [72] wrote that heating was performed in his series of patients using "temperatures of 42 °–43 °C". In a subsequent paper from the same group from the city of Hope National Center, California (Vora et al. [138]), more precise details are given. A thermistor is placed in the center of the treatment volume: it acts as a control for desired temperature and is not moved

during the whole hyperthermia session. Hyperthermia is given for 30–40 min with a "control temperature" of 42°–43 °C.

Manning, in one of the first Tucson papers [82], did not publish much detail about the temperature distributions which were obtained in the first 17 patients he treated (42.5°–43 °C). In a subsequent paper from the same group, Aristizabal and Oleson [3] gave more detailed results: temperature mapping was done by periodically translating thermometers by 1-cm increments through additionally implanted catheters. In their entire patient group (64 cases), the time-averaged maximum tumor temperature was 44.6 °C; the time-averaged minimum temperature was 41 °C. In their experience, it was difficult to achieve a minimum temperature above 41 °C.

The group in Birmingham, Alabama, reported very precise data concerning the temperature distribution they obtained in patients with lung cancers using the technique of "internal" (stainless steel filament woven through the tumor) and "external" (sheet of aluminum foil at the skin) electrodes. For the first patients Lilly et al. [77] reported the temperature as a function of time in three locations: in the lung tumor and in two different places in the normal lung, 2 cm outside the tumor. At the equilibrium (after 15 min), the authors were able to achieve 42 °C in the tumor, while the temperature did not exceed 39.6 °C in the normal surrounding lung.

In a subsequent paper from the same group (Brezovich [22]), the results of five patients were reported. The *maximum* tumor temperature (averaged over all ten hyperthermia treatments) was found to vary from patient to patient, being 42.5 °C, 45.9 °C, 41.6 °C, 40.9 °C and 42.9 °C, respectively. In contrast, the maximum temperature recorded in the normal lung varied to a smaller extent, from 36.9° to 38.3 °C.

Yabumoto and Suyama [143] in Japan, in seven patients, reported that they measured temperatures from 41° to 43 °C in a thermometer inserted in the tumor. They apparently only measured the temperature in two points: tumor and surrounding tissue.

Bicher et al. [12, 13] only reported that the tumor temperature is "maintained at 42–45 °C" without giving any data allowing an assessment of the precise temperature distribution within the tumor volume.

The group in Long Beach, California (Puthawala and Syed [107]), recently reported (in an abstract) that in 44 patients, tumors were heated between 42° and 43 °C, but no data about precise temperature distribution were available, either in this abstract or in a previous paper [106].

Borok and the group in Orange, New Jersey [17], also published an abstract on 20 patients treated with interstitial thermoradiotherapy for brain tumors. They reported that the patients were treated for 60 min at 43 °C: we can suppose that this temperature was recorded in the heating lines. It is understandable that in these brain tumor cases very precise thermal mapping by invasive methods could not be achieved.

The group in Villejuif, France [31, 34], has a machine which allows continuous recording of the temperature in all the heating lines. In most cases, one or several additional plastic catheters have been placed in the center of the tumor, in order to estimate the minimum tumor temperature within the heated volumes. Thus two parameters can be considered: first the "absolute" *minimum temperature*, secondly the *homogeneity* of the temperature distribution (e.g., the difference between the temperature in the heating probes – which is most likely to be the maximum temperature – and the minimum estimated temperature recorded in the additional catheters). For the 25 implantations for which such additional "thermometry" catheters have been placed and for which precise thermal mapping is available, a minimum temperature of 44 °C was attained in 16 cases (64%) and one of 43 °C in five cases (i.e., a minimum temperature of at least 43 °C was attained in 84% of the cases); a minimum temperature of only 42 °C was achieved in four cases. For the last nine patients, for whom we could not reach the prescribed minimum temperature of 44 °C, it would have been theoretically possible to overcome the problem by increasing the heating probe temperature to 47°–48 °C. However, such an increase in the probe temperatures would probably have led to burns or areas of necrosis. Moreover, for nonanesthesized patients, a temperature of 45.5°–46 °C in the heating probes was found to be highly uncomfortable.

If, as previously stated, the "inhomogeneity" of the temperature distribution is defined as the difference between the "hot" points (usually in the heating lines) and the "cold" points (usually recorded in the additional plastic tubes), the Villejuif group found that in 16 of the 25 evaluable implantations, inhomogeneity was less than (or equal to) 1 °C and that in 11 of these cases the inhomogeneity was 0 °C (mostly in small tumors). In eight cases inhomogeneities of between 2° and 3 °C were observed, and in one case an inhomogeneity of 4 °C was recorded (42 °C minimum temperature, with 46 °C in the heating probes).

The failure to reach a minimum prescribed temperature of 44 °C, or the lack of temperature homogeneity, could be attributed in this series to "incorrect" geometry of the implantation in a few cases. More often, unsatisfactory heating was observed despite an apparently "correct" implantation. In one case, an inhomogeneity of 2.5 °C could be attributed to the proximity of the temporal artery, but in the other cases it could only be supposed that local variations of blood flow and/or of tissue conductivities caused the observed temperature inhomogeneity.

Three French centers (Villejuif, Lyon, Dijon) recently reported the results of an interstitial thermoradiotherapy collaborative study [37]. Precise thermal mapping was available for 65 patients. A minimum temperature of 43 °C could be reached in 53 patients (81% of the cases), thus confirming the initial results obtained in Villejuif.

The group in St. Louis, Missouri (Emami et al. [52–55]), also underlined the need for additional catheters (minimum of two and maximum of six) to be placed in suitable positions for thermometry. In each treatment, the locations of maximum and minimum temperature were determined by mapping along the respective catheter tracks. Temperatures were recorded every 2 min until the desired temperature equilibrium was reached. This was then repeated every 10 min during the course of each hyperthermia session. Emami [55] considered a hyperthermia session satisfactory if the entire gross tumor volume was included in the implanted volume with clinically acceptable margins, *and* if the minimum tumor temperature was above 42 °C. With this definition, 37 lesions (out of 48: 77%) received a satisfactory hyperthermia treatment. Although the definition of "satisfactory heating" was slightly different, the results obtained here were similar to those achieved in the French centers.

In his experience, Linares [78] stated that homogeneous heat deposition is not always easily achieved. This is perhaps due to the size of the tumors he treated, i.e., large lesions from 30 to 1232 cc. Moreover, he was able to measure the temperature in 16 different points, thus obtaining good thermal mapping throughout these large volumes.

All these results suggest that a "satisfactory" heating (minimum temperature of at least 43 °C, acceptable homogeneity of the temperature distribution, heated volume encompassing the tumor with clinically acceptable margins) can be achieved with the presently available interstitial hyperthermia machines in about two-thirds of cases. This appears superior to what can be usually achieved with the classical external hyperthermia techniques (but the indications are obviously different).

On the other hand, some precise guidelines should be formulated concerning the way the thermometry data have to be reported. As previously underlined, the main temperature to be taken into account is the minimum temperature achieved in the heated volume. Since spatial resolution of noninvasive thermometry is still unsatisfactory (about 1 cm), the minimum temperature should be estimated by mapping along additionally implanted catheters, located at the center of the applications. In addition, data concerning the homogeneity of the temperature distribution are necessary. In anesthetized patients, a minimum temperature of 44 °C may be achieved, but with 48 °C, for example, in the heating probes; the risk of severe complications (burns, necrosis) is obviously higher in such patients than if the heating probe temperature has not exceeded 45 °C. Thus not only the minimum temperature, but also an assessment of the temperature homogeneity should be recorded. Lastly, as emphasized by Emami [55], we must make sure that the heated volume really encompasses the tumor mass, with "classical" safety margins.

1.3.6 Clinical Results

In this section, we shall first review the clinical results which have been reported so far by the different centers. The possible relationships between tumor response and treatment parameters (such as site and volume of the tumor, temperature level, and radiation dose) will be considered. We shall finally discuss the long-term clinical results of the interstitial hyperthermia–brachytherapy combination technique.

Only published papers where more than five patients were reported will be considered, whatever the technique used (RF or microwaves).

Vora et al. [138] treated 16 locally advanced malignant tumors. Six patients presented with breast cancers, three with uterine cervix tumors, two with rectal cancers, and there were five miscellaneous implanted sites, mainly superficial secondary tumors. For five lesions, the only previous "treatment" was a biopsy. The 11 other lesions received various treatments. Of these, six were previously irradiated, receiving doses in the range 48–80 Gy. Among the 15 evaluable treated tumors, 11 achieved a complete response, one a partial response (regression superior to 50%), and three showed no response. The same group recently published an abstract specifically dealing with 19 patients with advanced cancers of the cervix who received a pelvic implantation for interstitial thermoradiotherapy, but no precise clinical results were given [139].

In the review of the University of Arizona human clinical hyperthermia experience, Oleson et al. [94] reported on 163 patients treated with diverse techniques. Of these, 52 were treated by means of an interstitial hyperthermia–brachytherapy combination. These tumors were recurrent lesions after prior therapy, were judged unlikely to respond to conventional therapy, were accessible for thermometry, and the patients had a life expectancy superior to 6 months. Details of the tumor sites were not given. Among these 52 lesions, 20 showed complete response, 22 a partial response, and 10 no response.

Strohbehn et al. [127] reported six patients treated by an interstitial thermoradiotherapy technique. Except for one patient, it is not clear whether they received any previous irradiation. They observed three complete responses and two partial responses, while one patient did not respond.

Yabumoto and Suyama [143] published on seven patients. It was only stated that the lesions were "advanced accessible tumors," without any detail about possible previous treatments. They noted one complete and two partial responses; four patients were nonresponders.

Bicher et al. [13] treated eight patients using a sophisticated combination of external irradiation, interstitial irradiation, and hyperthermia (see Sect. 1.3.4). They reported five complete responses, two partial responses, and one nonresponder.

Cosset et al. [34], in the last update of the Institut Gustave-Roussy results, reported 29 lesions treated by interstitial thermoradiotherapy. Selection of the patients for this combination treatment was based on the failure to achieve local control of a tumor with conventional therapies. All the patients had previously received various combinations of radiation, surgery, and chemotherapy. Among the 23 patients (with 29 implanted lesions) of the series, 20 had received irradiation to a dose of at least 45 Gy to the site where interstitial thermoradiotherapy was subsequently given (three patients had received two "complete" courses of irradiation, to a total dose of 90–100 Gy). Among 23 evaluable lesions, 19 complete responses and four partial responses were observed. Recently, the data from Villejuif have been pooled with those of the Lyon and Dijon groups, in a French collaborative study (Cosset et al. [37]). Seventy-three lesions were treated: 21 cutaneous and/or subcutaneous metastatic lesions from various primaries (mainly breast cancers), 18 pelvic tumors (9 rectum and 9 uterus cancers), 18 recurrent head and neck tumors (mostly tongue cancers), 7 recurrent metastatic cervical nodes, 8 recurrent squamous cell carcinomas of the skin, and 1 penis cancer. Of 57 evaluable patients, 45 achieved a complete remission, 7 a partial remission, and there were 5 nonresponders.

Linares et al., at the Memorial Cancer Center in New York [78], treated ten advanced lesions of miscellaneous origin (four melanomas, three breast carcinomas, and one renal cell, one lung, and one gallbladder carcinoma). Three patients achieved complete tumor response and seven a partial response. However, two of these patients with partial response underwent a local excision of the persistent tumor mass after treatment, and no viable tumor was found on histological examination. Therefore we shall consider five complete and five partial responses in this series.

Puthawala et al., in Long Beach, California [106], treated a total of 43 patients with recurrent cancers of various sites (20 head and neck lesions, 13 pelvic tumors, and 10 lesions from miscellaneous origins). All lesions responded to the thermoradiotherapy combination. Complete tumor regression was noted in 37 patients (86%) within the first 6 months. In a subsequent abstract, the same authors reported 44 patients in a homogeneous series of recurrent and/or persistent squamous cell carcinoma of the head and neck. They observed a complete tumor response in 36 patients (82%), almost exactly confirming the results of their previous paper [107]. The same group recently published an abstract specifically dealing with the 39 patients with recurrent pelvic malignancies who had received a combination of interstitial irradiation and hyperthermia at the center since 1983. Overall local tumor control was achieved in 27 of 39 patients (69%) [131].

In the last update of the experience of the group of St. Louis, Missouri, Emami et al. [55] reported on 48 recurrent/persistent tumors in 46 patients, treated by interstitial thermoradiotherapy (with either RF or microwaves). The implanted sites included head and neck (29 cases), breast (6 cases), pelvis (7 cases) and 6 miscellaneous sites. All patients had failed extensive previous treatments. Radiation therapy had been previously given to most of the patients (45 cases). Among 44 evaluable lesions in this series, Emami reported 26 complete responses, 12 partial responses, and no response in 6 cases.

Recently, Lam et al. [74a] published their results for 31 recurrent of persistent tumors: they reported 19 complete, 11 partial responses and only one failure.

When pooling all these clinical data (Table 1.2) the total number of evaluable patients treated by interstitial thermoradiotherapy in the literature is to date 273. This number is an underestimate, since, for example, we only considered here the detailed paper of the Long Beach Group [106], and not the two subsequents abstracts [107, 131] from this center. In this total series, complete response was achieved in 172 cases (63%), partial response in 70 cases (26%), and no response 31 cases (11%). This is in good agreement with the previous attempts at evaluating the clinical efficacy of this combination technique by pooling data from the literature. Cosset [28], taking into account

Table 1.2. Clinical results thus far reported

Authors	Number of evaluable patients	Complete tumor response	Partial tumor response	No tumor response	Follow-up (months)
Vora et al. (1982) [138]	15	11	1	3	1–13
Oleson et al. (1984) [94]	52	20	22	10	3–18
Strohbein et al. (1984) [127]	6	3	2	1	Short
Yabumoto and Suyama (1984) [143]	7	1	2	4	2–13
Bicher et al. (1984) [13]	8	5	2	1	–
Puthawala et al. (1985) [106]	43	37	6	–	6
Cosset et al. (1986) [37]	57	45	7	5	2
Linares et al. (1986) [78]	10	5	5	–	Short
Emami et al. (1986) [55]	44	26	12	6	6–48
Lam et al. (1988) [74a]	31	19	11	1	1–24
Total	273	172 63%	70 26%	31 11%	

all the results which were presented at the 4th International Symposium on Hyperthermic Oncology (Aarhus, Denmark, 1984), reported a complete response rate of 65%, and a partial response rate of 18%. Emami et al. [55] considered separately the results obtained by the RF technique and those which were achieved by microwaves. In the RF series, they found a complete response rate of 51% and a partial response rate of 27%. In the microwave series, they reported a 63.5% complete response rate and a 25% partial response rate.

In the following sections, we shall study whether the clinical results (in fact the achievement of a complete remission) can be significantly related to some precise parameters.

1.3.6.1 Influence of Tumor Site

When considering the previous data, we find that almost half the patients treated by interstitial thermoradiotherapy presented with head and neck tumors (head and neck primary tumors and metastatic cervical lymph nodes). In the other half of the cases, there were approximately equal numbers of breast cancers, pelvic tumors (mainly cervical and rectal cancers), and miscellaneous sites (mostly superficial lesions).

Most of the patients presented with relapses in previously irradiated sites, even if the previously delivered doses were not always precisely specified.

The detailed analysis of the data presented in the previous section does not show any clear correlation between tumor site (or histology) and the achievement of a complete response. Only Oleson et al. [94], at Tucson, reported that within the group of 52 patients heated with the interstitial technique the complete response (CR) rate did vary significantly with site, with a P value of 0.012. However, the tumor site is strongly correlated with both tumor size and accessibility (and this accessibility is obviously a main parameter of the quality of hyperthermia). Moreover, the St. Louis results (Emami et al. [55]) suggest that neither histology nor tumor site has any significant impact on the final outcome.

Finally, we assume that tumor site has an impact on CR rate only because of its relationship with volume and accessibility. For example, the implanted cutaneous and/or subcutaneous nodules developing in the chest wall after previous irradiation for a breast cancer are often rather small and are mostly easily accessible for implantation. Better results are likely to be achieved in such cases than in an extended pelvic tumor for example.

1.3.6.2 Influence of Tumor Volume

There is general agreement that the tumor volume is one of the main parameters for achievement of a complete tumor response after interstitial thermoradiotherapy treatment.

The CR rate obtained by the Villejuif group (83%) (Cosset et al. [34]) is one of the best in the literature, but, at least for the first 14 patients of the series, the volume of the treated tumor was rather small (average tumor volume of 30 cc [31]). Conversely, the results of Linares et al. [78] showed a CR rate of "only" 50%, but they dealt with large tumor volumes, ranging from 30 to 1232 cc.

The Tucson group (Oleson et al. [94]) carefully analyzed their data and found that the CR rate did vary

significantly with tumor size ($P = 0.04$), the CR rate decreasing as volume increased.
In St. Louis, Emami et al. [55] also found that tumor size appeared to affect the tumor response. Of 13 tumors of less than 4 cm in average dimension, ten (77%) showed a complete response. Of 32 tumors with an average dimension of 4–10 cm, only 14 (44%) showed a complete response.
However, we must keep in mind that tumor size obviously governs the quality of the temperature distribution within the heated volume: the smaller the volume, the easier the achievement of a satisfactory hyperthermia session. The respective importance of these two parameters has yet to be determined.

1.3.6.3 Influence of the Quality of Hyperthermia

In one of the first reviews of the literature data, published in 1984, Aristizabal and Oleson [3] underlined the role of the temperature distribution in achieving a complete tumor response. In particular, they noted that the consistently high minimum temperature (44 °C) which could be achieved in most of the patients in the first Villejuif series (Cosset et al. [31]) translated into a significant increase in CR rate relative to other studies. The Villejuif group later reported that among the four partial regressions observed in a subsequent series [33], three were cases in which a satisfactory minimum temperature could not be obtained.
Oleson et al. [94], reviewing the Tucson data, found that the CR rate varied significantly with the minimum temperature achieved in the first hyperthermia treatment ($P = 0.013$) and in all the hyperthermia treatments, when several sessions were given ($P = 0.003$).
Emami et al. [55] considered separately 37 patients receiving at least one "statisfactory" hyperthermia session (for definition see Sect. 1.3.5) and 11 patients for whom no satisfactory hyperthermia session could be given. Among the 37 patients with "satisfactory" heating, there were 26 complete responses (70%), seven partial responses, three nonresponders, and one unknown result. In the 11 patients with no satisfactory hyperthermia session, no complete response was observed, and only five partial responses. This difference was satistically significant ($P = 0.001$).
In addition to these human data, it is interesting to recall that a statistically significant correlation between the minimum temperature achieved in the treated volume and the CR rate was shown by Dewhirst et al. [44] in spontaneous animal tumors.
As could be expected, the "quality", of the hyperthermia treatment thus appears to be a major parameter for achievement of a complete tumor response.

1.3.6.4 Influence of the Combined Radiation Dose

Since the combined radiation doses varied to a large extent from center to center and often within a given study, the evaluation of the role of the radiation dose in the CR rate is not easy. However, some data are available: at Villejuif, a dose of 30 Gy (brachytherapy) was given in the first 17 implantations. The immediate results were satisfactory [34], but two local relapses were observed. The dose was increased to 40 Gy for the subsequent implantations (and occasionally to 50 Gy), and no local relapse was noted.
At Tucson, Oleson et al. [94] found a statistically significant correlation between the CR rate and radiation dose, with a P value of 0.02.
Therefore, a "low" combined radiation dose could lead to a poor CR rate and/or local relapses, even after a complete regression of the tumor has been obtained.
The definition of the optimal combined radiation dose is still difficult. It seems advisable not to decrease the dose below 30–40 Gy. Conversely, a "high" combined dose could lead to severe complications (depending on the amount of previous irradiation). For previously treated areas, it seems wise not to exceed 40–45 Gy. For areas not previously treated, as stated above, the classical radiation dose could be given.

1.3.6.5 Respective Impact of the Different Parameters on Clinical Results

We previously emphasized that most of the parameters which have been considered above are in fact closely linked to each other. It is therefore of interest to use logistic regression analysis to investigate the relative prognostic importance of the different variables that were found to be individually important.
For the patients treated by means of interstitial thermoradiotherapy, only the Tucson group presented such an analysis (Oleson et al. [94]). They reported that tumor volume ($P = 0.008$), radiation dose ($P = 0.002$), and patient's sex ($P = 0.031$) were the most important parameters in predicting response. Histology, age, and (a little surprisingly) temperature variables could not improve prediction in the models. Recently, the same group (Shimm et al. [117]) reported a multivariate analysis of the various predictors of

complete response and response duration, from a series of 244 patients treated using various techniques combining hyperthermia and radiation (of these, 66 were treated using interstitial techniques). They found that temperature achieved, tumor volume, and radiation dose were the most significant independent predictors of complete response, whereas tumor site, heating technique, and temperature were the most significant predictors of response duration.

1.3.6.6 Long-term Tumor Control

As emphasized by Aristizabal and Oleson [3], the present criteria for evaluation of tumor response (no response, partial or complete response) can be criticized from a clinical point of view. The best criterion would be "local control" of the malignant tumor. This local control cannot be equated with complete response. In an early series treated by interstitial hyperthermia alone at Villejuif (Cosset et al. [29]), the CR rate was high but most patients relapsed within the first 6 months.

Unfortunately, evaluation of long-term local control is difficult with the presently available data: for ethical reasons the clinicians who began to deal with interstitial thermoradiotherapy had to treat advanced tumors which had failed on previous treatments. In almost all the published series, the general condition of the patients was poor. A large number of patients died within a few months from distant metastases (which were not treated by the interstitial hyperthermia–brachytherapy combination) or even from intercurrent problems [33]. This usual short follow-up (see Table 1.2) made any precise evaluation of the long-term local control difficult.

Only a few papers give information about relapses after complete regression has been obtained. Out of 19 lesions for which complete remission was achieved, Cosset et al. [34] observed six relapses. In fact, four of them occurred at the *edges* of the treatment volume and were obviously related either to technical problems (few heating lines were initially available) and/or to an incorrect evaluation of the volume to be implanted, and not to a real failure of the combination technique. Two relapses occurred *in* the treated volume (we previously noted that these two patients received only 30 Gy in combination with interstitial hyperthermia). These two relapses occurred at 5 and 9 months, respectively. The total number of local relapses, as in most other series, may have been underestimated since five patients in the Villejuif series died (from causes other than local relapses) less than 9 months after treatment.

Puthawala et al. [106] observed five relapses among their 37 patients who initially achieved a complete remission. These relapses occurred more than 6 months after the treatment.

Emami et al. [55], reported three (local?) relapses in 26 complete responders, at 6, 9, and 11 months, respectively. This observed ratio and delay for relapse are in good agreement with the Villejuif and Long Beach data.

From the rare available data, we can speculate that a long-term tumor control could be obtained in 80%–90% of the patients achieving a complete regression, but more detailed studies are still warranted to settle this point.

1.3.7 Toxicity

Most of the patients who have been treated so far using the combination of interstitial hyperthermia and brachytherapy previously received some type of irradiation (see Sect. 1.3.6). Hence the only toxicity we are able to evaluate is the toxicity of the *combination* of a previous irradiation (to various doses) and interstitial thermoradiotherapy (considered as a salvage treatment).

A variety of complications have been reported: some were only minor lesions (entry point localized burns such as were reported early by Joseph et al. [72], or minor wounds with delayed healing [54]) but others were more severe (e.g., large necrotic craters, orocutaneous or vesicovaginal fistulae [94]).

In their series of 16 lesions, Vora et al. [138] reported only three complications (19%). Two were local thermal burns at the implant site, both healing completely within 1 month. The last complication was a vesicovaginal fistula (i.e., a 6% severe complication rate).

Oleson et al. at Tucson utilized a toxicity score from 0 to 3 (0, no toxicity; 1, mild toxicity; 2, moderate toxicity; 3, severe toxicity) [94]. In fact this score was developed for all the different hyperthermia techniques and is better adapted to external than to interstitial hyperthermia. Anyway, the results deserve interest. For interstitially treated patients, the *severe* complications mainly consisted of fistulae between pelvic organs, mostly requiring surgical intervention. Out of the 52 lesions of the series, the authors reported ten complications score 1–3 (i.e., an overall ratio of 19%, exactly the same as reported by Vora et al. [138]). Of these, six (11%) were severe toxicity cases – score 3.

In the series of 29 implantations performed at the Institut Gustave-Roussy in Villejuif, Cosset et al. [34] reported 12 complications (41%). Eight were small areas of superficial necrosis, which usually took several months to heal completely, while four were large necrotic craters occurring rapidly (within a few weeks) in three cases and later (after a year) in one case. These four severe complications comprised two large superficial ulcerating skin lesions and two recurrent oral cavity tumors. The rate of severe complications was 14% in this series.

Puthawala et al. [106], in the Long Beach series, reported nine complications among 43 patients treated (21%). Of these, five could be considered severe lesions: one brachial neuropathy, two cases of necrosis of the vagina, and two enterovaginal fistulae. The rate of severe complications was 11%.

Linares et al. [78], at the Memorial Cancer Center of New York, noted four complications out of their ten treated lesions (overall complication rate: 40%). Of these, three were minor complications (mainly blisters occurring at the site of needle insertions) and did not require specific treatment. Only one patient developed a serious complication: this patient presented with a chest wall relapse of a previously irradiated breast cancer. After a combination of external irradiation and interstitial hyperthermia (for salvage treatment), rapid tumor necrosis developed, with persistent ulceration that did not heal with conservative treatment. A chest wall resection had to be performed; no viable tumor was found on the specimen. The rate of severe complications in this small series was 10%.

Emami et al. [55] carefully analyzed the complications in the series of 48 lesions they treated in St. Louis, Missouri. They reported 12 complications (overall complications rate: 25%). Of these, four could be considered minor: two cases of delayed wound healing and two of cutaneous sinus. Conversely, there were six cases of delayed healing necrotic craters (the result of rapid necrosis of large tumors), one orocuteneous fistula, and one vesicovaginal fistula. If these last eight cases are scored as "severe" complications, the rate of severe toxicity in this series was 17%.

Table 1.3 summarizes the data from the literature. The overall rate of complications ranges from 19% to 41%. The rate of severe complications ranges from 6% to 17%.

It is remarkable that the highest rate of toxicity (41%) was reported by the group who delivered the highest "thermal dose" and who obtained the highest rate of complete regression: the French group from Villejuif [34]. At least in cases of salvage treatment in previously irradiated areas, a significant level of complications appears to be the price to be paid for a high complete regression rate.

Moreover, a closer analysis of the data seems to indicate that some factors make some level of toxicity inevitable. The first predisposing factor is the amount of previous irradiation: the higher the dose which was previously delivered, the higher the risk of complications. The combination of interstitial hyperthermia and brachytherapy can be tolerated after a "classical" course of irradiation in most cases (i.e., a previous irradiation dose of 45–60 Gy). This same salvage combination is usually not tolerated after high dose previous irradiation or after two previous complete courses of radiotherapy.

Another factor in possible severe toxicity of interstitial thermoradiotherapy could be previous brachytherapy in the treated volume. Large necrotic craters have been noted in patients previously treated by external irradiations plus brachytherapy or by brachytherapy alone for tongue cancers, both in Villejuif (Cosset et al. [34]) and in St. Louis (Emami et al. [55]).

As could be expected, the rapid necrosis which was obtained after interstitial thermoradiotherapy of large ulcerating skin lesions often led to large necrotic craters. Emami et al. [55] and Cosset et al. [34] underlined the long healing time of these lesions (usually several months). In some cases, surgery had to be performed (Linares et al. [78], Cosset et al. [33]).

The last factor predisposing to severe complications is the presence of old scars. In Villejuif, when treating large volumes including a scar, necrosis was often spe-

Table 1.3. Data from the literature regarding complications

	Number of cases	All complications		Severe complications	
		(*n*)	(%)	(*n*)	(%)
Vora et al. (1982) [138]	16	3	19	1	6
Oleson et al. (1984) [94]	52	10	19	6	11
Cosset et al. (1985) [34]	29	12	41	4	14
Puthawala et al. (1985) [106]	43	9	21	5	11
Linares et al. (1986) [78]	10	4	40	1	10
Emami et al. (1986) [55]	48	12	25	8	17

cifically observed along the scar. The same observation has been made by the group in Lyon (J.P. Gerard, G. D. Laroche, personal communication) and in Dijon (J.C. Horiot, personal communication). This could be related to a higher conductivity of the scars "concentrating" the electric field. More likely, it is caused by a lower perfusion rate of the old scar tissues.

In conclusion, an overall complication rate of about 30%, with approximately 10% severe complications, as reported in the literature, can be regarded as acceptable when bearing in mind that this has been obtained in previously irradiated areas. These results suggest that in volumes *not* previously irradiated, a combination of normal radical dose irradiation and interstitial hyperthermia can be tolerated, provided that attention is paid to risk factors such as large ulcerating skin lesions and/or the presence of old scars in the treated volume. However, this should be unequivocally demonstrated in future series.

1.4 Future Prospects

1.4.1 Development of the Techniques

It can be reasonably expected that the various interstitial hyperthermia techniques will be improved in the next few years. The problems are clearly different for the radiofrequency method and for the microwave technique.

At present, the radiofrequency interstitial hyperthermia technique is ready for use. The generators are efficient, convenient, and reliable, and different machines are commercially available. Only some further refinements of the implantation material can be expected in the near future.

The microwave amplifiers are also ready and commercially available, but all the problems concerning the antennae have not yet been solved. Several groups are trying to overcome the main problem of the adaptation of the antenna's length to a given tumor, proposing different solutions. From what we know about the preliminary results, we can reasonably expect that the clinicians will have a more "adaptable" microwave technique available in the next 2 years (see Sect. 1.2.2).

The inductively heated ferromagnetic seeds are still under study. More than the technique itself, the precise indications for such an original method, with its advantages and drawbacks, need to be specifically defined.

1.4.2 The Search for New Indications: the Example of Interstitial Hyperthermia of Brain Tumors

Now that stereotactic techniques have enabled neurosurgeons to implant needles or catheters safely and precisely in the brain, interstitial irradiation of primary brain tumors has been proposed, either with iodine 125 sources held in catheters or with iridium 192 wires [11, 133]. Unfortunately, in spite of some encouraging preliminary results, such attempts have not significantly changed the normal poor prognosis of high grade gliomas [15]: tumor recurrences and radiation necrosis of normal brain tissue around the lesions have remained unsolved problems.

Thus, in an attempt to improve the prognosis of these tumors, the addition of interstitial hyperthermia to brain brachytherapy has been considered.

A group in San Francisco (Sneed et al. [118]) recently studied interstitial microwave hyperthermia in a canine brain model. They used dipole antennae working at 915 MHz and 2450 MHz, inserted in plastic catheters. In fact, as could be expected, 915-MHz antennae could not be inserted to the "ideal" depth of 8 cm in the dog brains; shorter 2450-MHz antennae (2 cm) were therefore chosen for the heating trials. The distribution of temperature which was observed around a single probe in the normal dog brain was what could be predicted from previous studies. The radial distribution of the temperature, perpendicular to the antenna junction, shows a 7 °C drop from 0 to 1 cm away from the probe. The authors defined a reference point located 0.5 cm radially away from the antenna junction, and maintained the temperature at 44 °C for 30 min at that point in four dogs. They specified that the maximum temperature obtained near the antenna junction was approximately 5 °C hotter than the "reference" temperature. (This means that a small volume immediately around the antenna received about 49 °C for 30 min). A first interesting observation was that a lower temperature was observed at the point where the probe passed through the longitudinal fissure. Thus it could be advisable to avoid implantation of the antennae perpendicular to the main brain sulci in human patients.

Secondly, the authors were able to study histological evidence of brain damage after such an application of interstitial hyperthermia given alone. The region which received more than 44 °C for 30 min (1 cm in diameter) showed a frank coagulation necrosis. This necrotic volume was surrounded by a sharply defined ring of damaged but apparently viable tissue. Furthermore, around this ring a variety of prominent vascular changes were observed. These three areas were clearly seen on control CT scans which were performed 1 week after hyperthermia.

Comparing the respective thermal and radiation brain injuries, the authors assumed that hyperthermia produces less extensive peripheral damage than does irradiation. Moreover, hyperthermia injuries appeared to evolve more rapidly. Obviously, the usual addition of irradiation to hyperthermia will alter the response of normal tissue to thermal injury, but these data give interesting guidelines for the clinical applications, showing the sensitivity of normal brain tissue to hyperthermia given at a therapeutic level. It seems that we cannot advise giving more than 44 °C for 30 min (or an equivalent thermal dose) either to a large brain volume or to an area responsible for major functions.

In contrast with these quite precise animal data, human clinical reports are still scarce and anecdotal [23, 79]. A group in Baltimore (Salcman, Samaras et al.), after presenting the biophysical rationale of their microwave technique [112], published detailed experimental studies [114, 115]. They then reported the results of a phase I trial, evaluating the technical feasibility and clinical safety of interstitial microwave hyperthermia in six patients with glioblastoma recurring after surgery, irradiation, and chemotherapy. After two hyperthermia treatments (45 °C for 60 min – reference point unspecified), four of the six patients have lived 18 months after implantation, two of them having negative CT scans at 18 and 27 months since recurrence [113].

Borok et al. in Orange, New Jersey [17], recently reported on 20 patients with biopsy-proven recurrent brain malignancies. All previously received brain irradiation. Fifteen patients received interstitial 2450 MHz microwave hyperthermia *alone* (43 °C for 60 min – reference point not specified). The other five patients, selected with more favorable performance status and no active malignancy elsewhere, received additional brachytherapy by iridium 192, to doses varying from 10 to 22.5 Gy after hyperthermia treatment. Among the 15 patients given hyperthermia alone, 12 objective responses (mass reduction and/or tumor necrosis) were observed. Of the five patients receiving the hyperthermia–brachytherapy combination, four showed an objective tumor response. More precision and follow-up are needed to confirm these first clinical data, and further studies are clearly required.

1.4.3 Intraoperative Interstitial Hyperthermia

A large number of medicosurgical teams are presently dealing with intraoperative radiotherapy, with some encouraging preliminary results [64, 88, 109]. Others have devoted their efforts toward the operative implantation of various materials (usually plastic tubes) to be secondarily afterloaded with radioactive seeds or wires [101]. It is thus understandable that some attention has been drawn to the possible use of "intraoperative interstitial hyperthermia," or, more exactly, to the intraoperative implantation of various catheters to be used as guides for subsequent interstitial hyperthermia.

In 1984, Frazier and Corry reported on 12 patients presenting with thoracic or abdominal tumors which were found to be unresectable at surgery. The electrodes were fashioned at the time of surgery and placed at the periphery of the tumor. High "average" temperature levels could be achieved. At the time of publication, only two patients were alive, one with a 6 month and one with a 3-year follow-up. Unfortunately, no details were available concerning the "adjuvant radiotherapy" which was given to the patients, and the precise evaluation of this series is difficult [60].

More recently, another group has reported on such an intraoperative attempt, publishing a short series of four patients (Coughlin et al. [41]). Actually the last patient in the series can hardly sustain the definition of "intraoperative" hyperthermia: this patient was treated for a recurrent carcinoma of the tongue and was given a classical implantation of plastic tubes under general anesthesia, as described in Sect. 1.3.1.3. The other three patients underwent laparotomy. On exploration, they were found to have persistent or recurrent unresectable tumor masses. The three lesions were implanted with plastic catheters. The authors underline the use of the "double lumen catheter" (one catheter overcoating the other), which appeared to reduce the risk of catheter kinking. A first hyperthermia session was given using microwave antennae inserted in the catheters after the patients recovered from surgery. Maximum temperature measured in the tumor reached 49 °C in one patient, but temperatures at the tumor margins were only in the range of 39–41 °C. Hyperthermia was given for 60 min. Immediately following hyperthermia, antennae and thermometry probes were removed and iridium 192 seeds afterloaded. The irradiation doses were in the range of 66–85 Gy (at the center of the volume). The seeds were then removed and a second 60-min hyperthermia treatment administered. The authors emphasized that hyperthermia treatments were not power limited by patient pain, probably because there are no, or few, thermal receptors at depth in the body. The patients in this study have remained free of recurrence for at least 6 months. The follow-up is too short to ensure that local control was obtained; moreover, the high brachytherapy dose which was delivered could account for the good tumor response. Anyway, this paper proves the feasibility of the technique, and this new approach could widely extend the frame of the indications for interstitial thermoradiotherapy.

1.4.4 The Need for Randomized Studies

The clinical results which have been reported so far by the various groups are obviously encouraging. A high rate of complete tumor regression could be achieved for malignant lesions recurring in previously irradiated fields; moreover some patients experienced long survivals without any local relapse, demonstrating that local control could be obtained in a significant proportion of cases.

Some authors underlined that lesions which were initially considered as ineligible for salvage brachytherapy could be efficiently treated by the interstitial hyperthermia–brachytherapy combination [34]. However, as emphasized in Aristizabal and Oleson's review [3], other groups have reported good results of brachytherapy *alone* for lesions relapsing in previously irradiated fields. Syed et al. [128] documented a 63% local control rate after brachytherapy in patients with persistent and/or recurrent head and neck carcinomas. Puthawala et al. [104, 105] reirradiated 90 patients with recurrent pelvic tumors, achieving local control in 67% of these cases, with a complication rate of 15%.

Actually, the different interstitial thermoradiotherapy nonrandomized studies, whose results were previously analyzed, are indeed promising, but they are unable to demonstrate unequivocally an advantage of interstitial thermoradiotherapy over brachytherapy alone.

After these necessary pilot studies, we clearly have now to think about randomized trials. There are two subsets of patients which can be considered for such trials: previously irradiated patients (who relapsed in previously treated areas) and those not previously treated.

The American Radiation Therapy Oncology Group (RTOG) has currently activated a prospective randomized study to evaluate the therapeutic impact of interstitial thermoradiotherapy versus brachytherapy alone for lesions which have relapsed in previously irradiated fields [55]. No results are available yet.

The "philosophy" of the European Society for Hyperthermic Oncology (ESHO) is slightly different. The European groups agree that interstitial thermoradiotherapy can be useful for relapsing lesions, but are reluctant to propose a randomized study for this type of tumor. Actually the different sites and sizes of these lesions, the usually poor life expectancy, the various previous treatments, and the possible contraindications (or limitations) to brachytherapy because of the amount of previously delivered irradiation will make difficult the analysis of such a study. Hence the European authors have chosen to concentrate on tumors not previously irradiated.

In these cases, it seems obvious that interstitial hyperthermia should *not* be combined with brachytherapy techniques presently yielding excellent local tumor control. The addition of hyperthermia would be unlikely to improve significantly a 95% local control rate, and might be (slightly) detrimental by increasing the side-effects. In addition we must keep in mind that a review of recent reports [3] covering several hundred patients reveals that the local control rates achieved with brachytherapy alone are usually in the range of 70%–100%, with an incidence of complications between 10% and 20%.

Thus a reasonable attitude should be to consider for the interstitial hyperthermia trials *only* tumors whose local control (achieved by brachytherapy alone or by a combination of external irradiation and brachytherapy) is significant, but still unsatisfactory. The best candidates would be tumors for which the usual local in control is in the range 40%–60%, since we could then expect a significant improvement control, possibly leading to an improvement in survival.

Among these tumors, base of the tongue cancers have been considered. The unsatisfactory survival rate is due to a failure of local control in a significant proportion of cases. Isolated nodal failures are rare, as are isolated distant metastases [68]. Most centers presently treat such patients using irradiation alone. The results reported by the authors using *external* irradiation alone vary from center to center: the control rate is usually in the range 30%–50% [16, 84, 141]. Actually in all series the local control rate is closely dependent on the local extent of the disease (T classification). This was well shown in a recent study at the Institut Curie [71]. The Houston group reported better results, but included tumors of the lateral pharyngeal wall [119].

In an effort to improve the local control, several groups have proposed combining *external irradiation* and *brachytherapy*. Preliminary results on small series reported by Syed et al. [128], Parsons et al. [99], and Goffinet et al. [63] were encouraging. In a nonrandomized study, Baillet et al. [8] found a definite advantage of the external – interstitial irradiation combination over external radiotherapy alone. In an unpublished series of 108 patients treated by an external irradiation – brachytherapy combination at Villejuif (Lusinchi et al.), the 5-year control rate was 65%.

In a large comparative but nonrandomized series treated at Nancy (Hoffstetter et al. [68]), a definite advantage in terms of local control and survival was found for the brachytherapy-external irradiation combination. The 3-year crude survival was 14% after external irradiation alone, and 45% after combined brachytherapy and external irradiation.

Thus the association of external irradiation and brachytherapy is being proposed for cancers of the base of the tongue in an increasing number of center. However, the control rates which have been reported should be improved: the addition of interstitial hyperthermia to this external and interstitial irradiation combination should be considered, in the hope of increasing the control rate (and possibly the survival) without adding much to the toxicity.

A European multicenter randomized study is presently under discussion to compare for primary tumors of the base of the tongue:

1. External irradiation (45 – 50 Gy) + brachytherapy (25 – 30 Gy)
2. The same external and interstitial irradiation combined with interstitial hyperthermia (43.5 °– 44 °C, 45 min, before brachytherapy)

1.5 Conclusions

In *A Treatise on Actinic-Ray Therapy* (mainly dealing with hyperthermia treatments), published in 1922, T.H. Plank [102] wrote "Remember once and for all time that these rays are not a panacea for all the ills of human flesh, but that they are ONE of the methods of treating these ills." With only slight changes, this assumption can still be applied to interstitial hyperthermia.

The basic rationale of hyperthermia has been settled enough to justify the present clinical studies. Among the different techniques, interstitial hyperthermia has proven to be one of the best methods of heating, when considering the levels of temperature which can be reached and the homogeneity of the temperature distribution. Large pilot studies in different centers throughout the world have shown the clinical efficacy of interstitial hyperthermia when combined with brachytherapy. Provided strict guidelines are respected, toxicity is acceptable.

The problem is now to define the exact role that interstitial hyperthermia should play in the anticancer armamentarium. We can reasonably expect that this role will be real at least in a small number of well-defined clinical situations, but we shall be able to specify it precisely only when we have the results of large multicenter randomized trials, such as that being undertaken in the United States under the auspices of the RTOG or that under discussion in Europe under the auspices of the ESHO.

Acknowledgments. The author would like to acknowledge the help of Michael Ashby and Paul Carnochan in the preparation of the manuscript.

References

1. Anghileri LJ, Robert J (1986) Hyperthermia in cancer treatment, vol 3. CRC, Boca Raton, Florida
2. Arcangeli G, Barni E, Cividalli A, Lovisolo G, Nervi C, Mauro F (1982) Hyperthermia by implantable applicators. In: Gautherie M, Albert E (eds) Biomedical thermology. Liss, New York, pp 641 – 647
3. Aristizabal SA, Oleson JR (1984) Combined interstitial irradiation and localized current field hyperthermia: results and conclusions from clinical studies. Cancer Res [Suppl] 44:4757 S-4760 S
4. Aristizabal S, Valencia A, Ocampo G, Surwit E (1986) Conventional intracavitary irradiation versus interstitial parametrial implants in carcinoma of the cervix stage IIIB (abstr). Int J Radiat Oncol Biol Phys 12 [Suppl 1]:94
5. Astrahan MA, George FW III (1980) A temperature regulating circuit for experimental localized current field hyperthermia systems. Med Phys 7:362 – 364
6. Astrahan MA, Norman A (1982) A localized current field hyperthermia system for use with 192 iridium interstitial implants. Med Phys 9:419 – 424
7. Atkinson WJ, Brezovich IA (1984) Interstitial heating of tumors by thermally self regulating nickel-copper seeds. Abstracts of the 4th international symposium of hyperthermic oncology, Aarhus, Denmark, July 2 – 6 (D10)
8. Baillet F, Deluen F, Delpon A, Housset M, Maylin C, Perret M (1983) La radiothérapie des épithéliomas de la base de langue. Actualités de cancérologie cervico-faciale 9:168 – 175
9. Ben-Hur E, Bronk BV, Elkind MM (1972) Thermally enhanced radiosensitivity of cultured Chinese hamster cells. Nature 238:209 – 211
10. Ben-Hur E, Elkind MM (1974) Thermally enhanced radioresponse of cultured Chinese hamster cells, damage and repair of single-stranded DNA and a DNA complex. Radiat Res 59(2):484 – 495
11. Bernstein M, Gutin PH (1981) Interstitial irradiation of brain tumors: a review. Neurosurgery 9:741 – 750

12. Bicher HI, Moore DW, Wolfstein RS (1984) A method for interstitial thermoradiotherapy. In: Overgaard J (ed) Hyperthermic oncology 1984, vol 1. Taylor and Francis, London, pp 595–598
13. Bicher HI, Wolfstein RS, Fingerhut AG, Frey HS, Lewinsky BS (1984) An effective fractionation regime for interstitial thermoradiotherapy–preliminary clinical results. In: Overgaard J (ed) Hyperthermic oncology 1984, vol 1. Taylor and Francis, London, pp 575–578
14. Bleehen NM (1985) Hyperthermia, the next stage in the oncologist's odyssey. In: Overgaard J (ed) Hyperthermic oncology 1984, vol 2. Taylor and Francis, London, pp 371–383
15. Bloom HJG (1982) Intracranial tumors: response and resistance to therapeutic endeavors 1970–1980. Int J Radiat Oncol Biol Phys 8:1083–1113
16. Blumberg AL, Fu KK, Phillips TL (1979) Results of treatment of carcinoma of the base of the tongue, the UCSF experience 1957–1976. Int J Radiat Oncol Biol Phys 5:1971–1976
17. Borok TL, Winter A, Laing J, Paglione R, Sterzer F, Sinclair I (1986) Microwave hyperthermia radiosensitized iridium 192 for recurrent brain malignancy (abstr). Int J Radiat Oncol Biol Phys 12 [Suppl 1]: 146
18. Bowman HF (1980) The bio-heat transfer equation and discrimination of thermally significant vessels. Ann NY Acad Sci 335:155–160
19. Bowman HF (1982) In: Nussbaum GH (ed) Physical aspects of hyperthermia. Am Inst Phys, New York, p 511
20. Breasted JH (1930) The Edwin Smith surgical papyrus. In: Licht S (ed) Therapeutic heat and cold, 2nd edn. Waverly, Baltimore, p 196
21. Brezovich IA, Atkinson WJ, Chakroborty DP (1984) Temperature distributions in tumor models heated by self-regulating nickel-copper alloy thermoseeds. Med Phys 11:145–152
22. Brezovich IA, Atkinson WJ, Lilly MB (1984) Local hyperthermia with interstitial techniques. Cancer Res [Suppl] 44:4752 S–4756 S
23. Britt RH, Lyons BE, Pounds DW, Prionas SD (1983) Feasibility of ultrasound hyperthermia in the treatment of malignant brain tumors. Med Instrum 17:172–177
24. Cetas TC (1982) Thermal dosimetry during hyperthermia. In: Gautherie M, Albert E (eds) Biomedical thermology. Liss, New York, pp 561–583
25. Cetas TC, Hevezi JM, Manning MR, Ozimek EJ (1982) Dosimetry of interstitial thermoradiotherapy. NCI Monogr 61:505–507
26. Chen MM (1982) In: Nussbaum GH (ed) Physical aspects of hyperthermia. Am Inst Phys, New York, p 549
27. Coley-Nauts H (1985) Hyperthermic oncology: historic aspects and future trends. In: Overgaard J (ed) Hyperthermic oncology 1984, vol 2. Taylor and Francis, London, pp 199–209
28. Cosset JM (1985) Interstitial techniques. In: Overgaard J (ed) Hyperthermic oncology 1984, vol 2. Taylor and Francis, London, pp 309–316
29. Cosset JM, Brule JM, Salama AM, Damia E, Dutreix J (1982) Low frequency (0.5 MHz) contact and interstitial techniques for clinical hyperthermia. In: Gautherie M, Albert E (eds) Liss, New York, pp 649–657
30. Cosset JM, Dutreix J, Damia E, Kantor G, Vannetzel JM, Gerbaulet A (1983) Distribution of temperature in volumes heated by interstitial hyperthermia (abstr). Strahlentherapie 159:369
31. Cosset JM, Dutreix J, Dufour J, Janoray P, Damia E, Haie C, Clarke D (1984) Combined interstitial hyperthermia and brachytherapy: Institute Gustave-Roussy technique and preliminary results. Int J Radiat Oncol Biol Phys 10:307–312
32. Cosset JM, Dutreix J, Gerbaulet A, Damia E (1984) Combined interstitial hyperthermia and brachytherapy: the Institute Gustave-Roussy experience. In: Overgaard J (ed) Hyperthermic oncology 1984, vol 1. Taylor and Francis, London, pp 587–590
33. Cosset JM, Dutreix J, Gerbaulet A, Damia E (1985) L'association hyperthermie interstitielle-curiethérapie: une technique de rattrapage des récidives en zones précédemment irradiées. In: Lemerle J (ed) Actualités carcinologiques de l'Institut Gustave-Roussy. Masson, Paris, pp 211–218
34. Cosset JM, Dutreix J, Haie C, Gerbaulet A, Janoray P, Dewar JA (1985) Interstitial thermoradiotherapy: a technical and clinical study of 29 implantations performed at the Institut Gustave-Roussy. Int J Hyperthermia 1:3–13
35. Cosset JM, Dutreix J, Lyonnard de la Girennerie O, Haie C, Janoray P, Horiot JC (1985) Resistive diathermy (0.5–1 MHz) for interstitial thermoradiotherapy: technique of implantation (abstr). Strahlentherapie 161:528
36. Cosset JM, Dutreix J, Haie C, Mabire JP, Damia E (1986) Technical aspects of interstitial hyperthermia. In: Bruggmoser G, Hinkelbein W, Engelhardt R, Wannenmacher M (eds) Locoregional high-frequency hyperthermia and temperature measurement. (recent results in cancer research, vol 101), Springer, Berlin, New York, Heidelberg, pp 56–60
37. Cosset JM, Gerard JP, Janoray P, Haie C, de Laroche G, Horiot JC, Dutreix J (1986) Advances in interstitial thermoradiotherapy (abstr). Proceedings of VIII meeting of hyperthermic oncology (ESHO), Tiberias, Israel, Sept 22–25, pp 61–62
38. Coughlin CT, Douple EB, Strohbehn JW, Eaton WL, Trembly BS, Wong TZ (1983) Interstitial hyperthermia in combination with brachytherapy. Radiology 148:285–288
39. Coughlin CT, Roberts DW, Wong TZ, Strohbehn JW, Douple EB, Colacchio TA (1984) Clinical experience with deep seated intra-abdominal and brain tumors using an interstitial microwave antenna array for hyperthermia. Abstracts of the 4th international symposium on hyperthermic oncology, Aarhus, Denmark, July 2–6 (D15)
40. Coughlin CT, Wong TZ, Guerkink N (1985) Implantation of maxillary antrum for delivery of iridium brachytherapy and microwave induced hyperthermia. Abstracts of the 33rd annual meeting of Rad Res Soc, Los Angeles, May 5–9, p 26
41. Coughlin CT, Wong TZ, Strohbehn JW, Colacchio TA, Sutton JE, Belch RZ, Douple EB (1985) Intraoperative interstitial microwave induced hyperthermia and brachytherapy. Int J Radiat Oncol Biol Phys 11:1673–1678
42. Deshmukh R, Damento M, Demer L, Forsyth K, Deyoung J, Dewhirst M, Cetas TC (1984) Ferromagnetic alloys with curie temperatures near 50 °C for use in hyperthermic therapy. In: Overgaard J (ed) Hyperthermic oncology 1984, vol 1. Taylor and Francis, London, pp 571–574
43. De Sieyes DC, Douple EB, Strohbehn JW, Trembly BS (1981) Some aspects of optimization of an invasive microwave antenna for local hyperthermia treatment of cancer. Med Phys 8:179–183
44. Dewhirst MW, Sim DA, Sapareto S, Connor WG (1984) The importance of minimum tumor temperature in deter-

mining early and long-term response of spontaneous pet animal tumors to heat and radiation. Cancer Res 44:43–50

45. Doss JD (1975) Use of RF fields to produce hyperthermia in animal tumors. In: Robinson JE (ed) Proceedings of the international symposium on cancer therapy by hyperthermia and radiation. American College of Radiology, Washington DC, p 226
46. Doss JD, McCabe CW (1976) A technique for localized heating in tissue: an adjunct to tumor therapy. Med Instrum 10:16–21
47. Double EB, Strohbehn JW, Bowers ED, Walsh JE (1979) Cancer therapy with localized hyperthermia using an invasive microwave system. J Microwave Power 14:181–186
48. Dutreix A, Marinello G, Wambersie A (1982) Dosimétrie en curiethérapie. Masson, Paris
49. Dutreix J, Damia E, Cosset JM, Salama M, Brule JM (1981) Techniques de chauffage pour l'hyperthermie. Bull Cancer (Paris) 68:240–248
50. Dutreix J, Cosset JM, Salama M, Brule JM, Damia E (1982) Experimental studies of various heating procedures for clinical application of localized hyperthermia. In: Gautherie M, Albert E (eds) Biomedical thermology. Liss, New York, pp 585–596
51. Dutreix J, Damia E, Salama AM, Janoray P, Cosset JM (1983) Rayonnement infra-rouge en hyperthermie thérapeutique. J Biophys Med Nucl 7:25–35
52. Emami B, Perez CA (1985) Interstitial thermoradiotherapy: an overview. Endocurie Hypertherm Oncol 1:35–40
53. Emami B, Marks JE, Perez CA, Nussbaum GH, Leybovich L, von Gerichten D (1984) Interstitial thermoradiotherapy in the treatment of recurrent/residual malignant tumors. Am J Clin Oncol 7:699–704
54. Emami B, Marks J, Perez C, Nussbaum G, Leybovich L (1985) Treatment of human tumors with interstitial irradiation and hyperthermia. In: Overgaard J (ed) Hyperthermic oncology 1984, vol 1. Taylor and Francis, London, pp 583–586
55. Emami B, Perez CA, Leybovich L, Straube W, von Gerichten D (1987) Interstitial thermoradiotherapy in treatment of malignant tumors. Int J Hyperthermia 3(2):107–118
56. Emery AF, Sekins KM (1982) In: Lehman JF (ed) Therapeutic heat and cold. Williams and Wilkins, Baltimore, p 133
57. Feder BH, Syed AMN, Neblett D (1978) Treatment of extensive carcinoma of the cervix with the "transperineal parametrial butterfly": a preliminary report on the revival of Waterman's approach. Int J Radiat Oncol Biol Phys 4:735–742
58. Fessenden P, Kapp DS, Schoeppel S, Samulski TV, Meyer J, Prionas SV, Lohrbach AW (1986) Local/regional hyperthermia of deep seated malignancies: a comparison of annular phased array microwave, focus ultrasound and interstitial RF devices (abstr). Int J Radiat Oncol Biol Phys 12 [Suppl 1]:153–154
59. Forsyth K, Deshmukh R, Deyoung DW, Dewhirst M, Cetas TC (1984) Recent clinical experience in pet animals with hyperthermic therapy in the head and neck region induced with inductively-heated ferromagnetic implants. In: Overgaard J (ed) Hyperthermic oncology 1984, vol 1. Taylor and Francis, London, pp 599–602
60. Frazier OH, Corry PM (1984) Induction of hyperthermia using implanted electrodes. Cancer Res [Suppl] 44:4864 S–4866 S
61. Gerner EW, Oval JH, Manning MR (1983) Dose rate dependence of heat radiosensitization. Int J Radiat Oncol Biol Phys 9:1401–1409
62. Gidman V, Roos D, Lindskoug BA (1984) Intercomparison of microwave antennas for hyperthermia. Abstracts of the 4th international symposium on hyperthermic oncology, Aarhus, Denmark, July 2–6 (D4)
63. Goffinet DR, Fee WE, Wells J, Austin-Seymour M, Clarke D, Mariscal JM, Goode RL (1985) Iridium 192 pharyngoepiglottic fold interstitial implants. The key to successful treatment of base tongue carcinoma by radiation therapy. Cancer 55: 941–948
64. Goldson AL (1981) Past, present and prospects of intraoperative radiotherapy (IOR). Semin Oncol 8:59–64
65. Hahn GM (1982) Hyperthermia and cancer. Plenum Press, New York
66. Hahn GM, Kernahan P, Martinez A, Pounds D, Prionas S, Anderson T, Justice G (1980) Some heat transfer problems associated with heating by ultrasound, microwaves or radiofrequency. In: Jain RK, Gullino PM (eds) Thermal characteristics of tumors: applications to detection and treatment. Ann NY Acad Sci 335:327
67. Harisiadis L, Sung D, Kessaris N, Hall EJ (1978) Hyperthermia and low dose rate irradiation. Radiology 129:195–198
68. Hoffstetter, S, Malissard L, Forcard JJ, Pernot M (1986) Carcinome épidermoïde de la base de langue. A propos de 108 cas traités au Centre Alexis Vautrin. J Eur Radiother 7:101–110
69. Jain RK (1983) In: Storm FK (ed) Hyperthermia in cancer therapy. Hall Medical, Boston MA, p 9
70. Janoray P, Horiot JC, Isturiz J, Chomono R, Cosset JM (1985) Interstitial hyperthermia and brachytherapy: experimental study on intestinal adenocarcinoma transplanted in the rat: preliminary results (abstr). Strahlentherapie 161:537
71. Jaulerry C, Bataini JP, Brunin F, Rodriguez J, Brugere J (1985) Facteurs pronostiques et résultats de l'irradiation externe des cancers de la base de langue. Ann Otolaryngol Chir Cervicofac 102:519–524
72. Joseph CD, Astrahan M, Lipsett J, Archambeau J, Forell B, George FW (1981) Interstitial hyperthermia and interstitial iridium 192 implantation: a technique and preliminary results. Int J Radiat Oncol Biol Phys 7: 827–833
73. Kantor G, Vannetzel JM, Dutreix J, Cosset JM, Damia E (1983) Infrared radiation in clinical hyperthermia (abstr). Strahlentherapie 159:377
74. Lagendijk JJW (1984) A new theory to calculate temperature distributions in tissues. In: Overgaard J (ed) Hyperthermic oncology 1984, vol 1. Taylor and Francis, London, p 507

74a. Lam K, Astrahan M, Langholz B, Jepson J, Cohen D, Luxton G, Petrovich Z (1988) Interstitial thermoradiotherapy for recurrent or persistent tumors. Int J Hyperthermia 4:259–266

75. Le Bourgeois JP, Convert G, Dufour J (1978) An interstitial device for microwave hyperthermia of human tumors. In: Streffer C (ed) Cancer therapy by hyperthermia and radiation. Urban & Schwarzenberg, Baltimore, pp 122–124
76. Lee DJ, O'Neill MJ, Lam KS, Rostock R, Lam WC (1986) A new design of microwave interstitial applications for hyperthermia with improved treatment volume. Int J Radiat Oncol Biol Phys 12:2003–2008
77. Lilly MB, Brezovich IA, Atkinson W, Chakraborty D, Durant JR, Ingram J, McElvein R (1983) Hyperthermia

with implanted electrodes. In vitro and in vivo correlations. Int J Radiat Oncol Biol Phys 9:373–382
78. Linares LA, Nort D, Brenner H, Shiu M, Ballon D, Anderson L, Alfieri A, Brennan M, Fucs Z, Hilaris B (1986) Interstitial hyperthermia and brachytherapy: a preliminary report. Endocurie Hypertherm Oncol 2:39–44
79. Lyons BE, Britt RH, Strohbehn JW (1984) Localized hyperthermia in the treatment of malignant brain tumors using an interstitial microwave antenna array. IEEE Trans Biomed Eng 31:53–62
80. Manning MR, Gerner EW (1983) Interstitial thermoradiotherapy. In: Storm FK (ed) Hyperthermia in cancer therapy. Hall, Boston, pp 467–478
81. Manning MR, Cetas TC, Gerner EW (1982) Interstitial thermoradiotherapy. NCI Monogr 61:357–360
82. Manning MR, Cetas TC, Miller RC, Oleson JR, Connor WG, Gerner EW (1982) Clinical hyperthermia: results of a phase I trial employing hyperthermia alone or in combination with external beam. Cancer 49:205–216
83. Marchal C, Hoffstetter S, Bey P, Pernot M, Gaulard ML (1985) Development of a new interstitial method of heating which can be used with conventional afterloading brachytherapy techniques using IR 192 (abstr). Strahlentherapie 161:543
84. Marcial VA, Hanley JA, Hendrickson F, Ortiz H (1983) Split course radiation therapy of carcinoma of the base of the tongue: results of a prospective national collaborative clinical trial conducted by the radiation oncology group. Int J Radiat Oncol Biol Phys 9:437–443
85. Martinez A, Schray MF (1986) Template and other extended techniques for pelvic and perineal implants (abstr). Int J Radiat Oncol Biol Phys 12 [Suppl 1]:84
86. Martinez A, Edmundson GK, Cox RS, Gunderson LL, Howes AE (1985) Combination of external beam irradiation and multiple site perineal applicator (MUPIT) for treatment of locally advanced or recurrent prostatic, anorectal and gynecologic malignancies. Int J Radiat Oncol Biol Phys 11:391–398
87. Matloubieh AY, Roemer RB, Cetas TC (1984) Numerical simulation of magnetic induction heating of tumors with ferromagnetic seed implants. IEEE Trans Biomed Eng 31:227–234
88. Mazeron JJ, Le Bourgeois JP, Ganem G (1986) La radiothérapie per-opératoire des tumeurs cancéreuses: passé, présent, perspectives. J Eur Radiother 7:1–14
89. Mechling JA, Strohbehn JW (1986) A theoretical comparison of the temperature distribution produced by three interstitial hyperthermia systems. Int J Radiat Oncol Biol Phys 12:2137–2142
90. Miller EC, Leith JT, Voemett RC, Gerner EW (1978) Effects of interstitial radiation therapy alone, or in combination with localized hyperthermia on a response of a mouse mammary tumor. J Radiat Res Tokyo 19:175–180
91. Nussbaum GH (1982) Physical aspects of hyperthermia. Am Inst of Phys, New York
92. Nussbaum GH, Leybovich L, Emami B, Perez CA (1982) Interstitial hyperthermia with multiplanar electrodes (abstr). Int J Radiat Oncol Biol Phys 8 (Suppl 1]:99
93. Nussbaum GH, Leybovich LB, Emami B, Perez CA, Johnston R, Straube WL (1984) Techniques for improved administration of interstitial hyperthermia with microwaves. Abstracts of the 4th international symposium of hyperthermic oncology, Aarhus, Denmark, July 2–6 (D3)
94. Oleson JR, Manning MR, Sim DA, Heusinkveld RS, Aristizabal SA, Cetas TC, Hevezi JM, Connor WG (1984) A review of the University of Arizona human clinical hyperthermia experience. Front Radiat Ther Oncol 18:136–143
95. Overgaard J (1984) Hyperthermic oncology 1984, vol 1. Proceedings of the 4th international symposium on hyperthermic oncology, Aarhus, Denmark, 2–6 July, Taylor and Francis, London
96. Overgaard J (1985) History and heritage. An introduction. In: Overgaard J (ed) Hyperthermic oncology 1984, vol 2. Taylor and Francis, London, pp 3–8
97. Overgaard J (1986) ESHO clinical protocols (abstr). Proceedings of VIIIth meeting of hyperthermic oncology (ESHO), Tiberias, Israel, Sept 22–25, p 41
98. Ozimek EJ, Cetas TC (1982) Thermal dosimetry during hyperthermia. NCI Monogr 61:509–512
99. Parksons JT, Million RR, Cassisi NJ (1982) Carcinoma of the base of the tongue. Results of radical irradiation with surgery reserved for irradiation failure. Laryngoscope 92:689–696
100. Perez CA, Emami B (1985) A review of current clinical experience with irradiation and hyperthermia. Endocurie Hypertherm Oncol 1:265–277
101. Pierquin B, Wilson JF, Chassagne D (1987) Modern brachytherapy. Masson, New York
102. Plank TH (1922) A treatise on actinic-ray therapy. Brown, Press. Munroe and Southworth, Chicago
103. Prionas SD, Goffinet DR, Samulski TV, Fessenden P, Hahn GM (1984) Characterization of an interstitial hyperthermia rf system utilizing flexible electrodes. Abstract of the 32nd annual meeting of Rad Res Soc, Orlando FL, March 25–29, p 14
104. Puthawala AA, Syed AMN, Fleming PA, Disaia PJ (1982) Reirradiation with interstitial implant for recurrent pelvic malignancies. Cancer 50:2810–2814
105. Puthawala AA, Syed AMN, Gates TC, McNamara C (1983) Integrated external and interstitial radiation therapy for primary carcinoma of the vagina. Obstet Gynecol 62:367–372
106. Puthawala AA, Syed N, Khalid MA, Rafie S, McNamara CS (1985) Interstitial hyperthermia for recurrent malignancies. Endocurie Hypertherm Oncol 1:125–131
107. Puthawala AA, Syed N, Khalid MA, Rafie S (1986) Thermoendocurietherapy for recurrent and/or persistent head and neck cancers (abstr). Int J Radiat Oncol Biol Phys 12 [Suppl 1]:110
108. Reinhold HS, Endrich B (1986) Tumor micro-circulation as a target for hyperthermia. Int J Hyperthermia 2:111–137
109. Rich TA (1986) Intra-operative radiotherapy. Radiother Oncol 6:207–221
110. Roos D (1984) Analysis of the temperature distribution produced by an invasive microwave applicator for heat treatment of cancer. Presented at the 4th international symposium of hyperthermia oncology, Aarhus, Denmark, July 2–6
111. Roos D, Hamnerius Y (1984) Development of a microwave applicator for intra-cavitary hyperthermia treatment. Abstracts of the 4th international symposium on hyperthermic oncology, Aarhus, Denmark, July 2–6 (D6)
112. Salcman M, Samaras GM (1981) Hyperthermia for brain tumors: biophysical rationale. Neurosurgery 9:327–335
113. Salcman M, Samaras GM (1983) Interstitial microwave hyperthermia for brain tumors: results of a phase-I clinical trial. J Neuro Oncol 1:225–236
114. Samaras GM (1984) Intracranial microwave hyperthermia: heat induction and temperature control. IEEE Trans Biomed Eng 31:63–69

115. Samaras GM, Salcman M, Cheung AY, Abdo HS, Schepp RS (1982) Microwave-induced hyperthermia: an experimental adjunct for brain tumor therapy. NCI Monogr 61:477–482
116. Sapozink MD, Palos B, Goffinet DR, Hahn GM (1983) Combined continuous ultra-low dose rate irradiation and radiofrequency hyperthermia in the C3H mouse. Int J Radiat Oncol Biol Phys 9:1357–1365
117. Shimm D, Cetas T, Sim D, Fletcher A, Bryson M, Gerner E, Cassady JR (1986) Hyperthermia in the treatment of human cancers (abstr). Int J Radiat Oncol Biol Phys 12 [Suppl 1]:153
118. Sneed PK, Matsumoto K, Stauffer P, Fike JR, Smith V, Gutin PH (1986) Interstitial microwave hyperthermia in a canine brain model. Int J Radiat Oncol Biol Phys 12:1887–1897
119. Spanos WJ, Shukovsky LJ, Fletcher GH (1976) Time, dose and tumor volume relationship in irradiation of squamous cell carcinomas of the base of the tongue. Cancer 37:2591–2599
120. Stauffer PR, Cetas TC, Jones RC (1982) System for producing localized hyperthermia in tumors through magnetic induction heating of ferromagnetic implants. NCI Monogr 61:483–487
121. Strohbehn JW (1983) Temperature distributions from interstitial RF electrode hyperthermia systems: theoretical predictions. Int J Radiat Oncol Biol Phys 9:1655–1667
122. Strohbehn JW, Douple EB (1985) Hyperthermia and cancer therapy: a review of biomedical engineering contributions and challenges. IEEE Trans Biomed Eng 32:779–787
123. Strohbehn JW, Mechling JA (1986) Interstitial techniques for clinical hyperthermia. In: Hand JW, James JR (eds). Physical techniques in clinical hyperthermia. Wiley, New York, pp 210–287
124. Strohbehn JW, Bowers ED, Walsh JE, Douple EB (1979) An invasive microwave antenna for locally-induced hyperthermia for cancer therapy. J Microwave Power 14:339–350
125. Strohbehn JW, Trembly BS, Douple EB (1982) Blood flow effects on the temperature distributions from an invasive microwave antenna array used in cancer therapy. IEEE Trans Biomed Eng 29:649–661
126. Strohbehn JW, Trembly BS, Douple EB, De Sieyes DC (1982) Evaluation of an invasive microwave antenna system for heating deep-seated tumors. NCI Monogr 61:489–491
127. Strohbehn JW, Douple EB, Coughlin CT (1984) Interstitial microwave antenna array systems for hyperthermia. Front Radiat Ther Oncol 18:70–74
128. Syed AMN, Feder BH, George FW (1977) Afterloading interstitial implant in the treatment or oral cavity and oropharyngeal cancers. Radiol Clin North Am 46:390–397
129. Syed AMN, Puthawala A, Neblett D, George FW III, Myint US, Lipsett JA, Jackson BR, Flemming PA (1978) Primary treatment of carcinoma of the lower rectum and anal canal by a combination of external irradiation and interstitial implant. Radiology 128:199–203
130. Syed AMN, Puthawala AA, Lansey LA, Shanberg AM, Neblett D, McNamama C (1983) Temporary iridium 192 implantation in the management of carcinoma of the prostate. In: Hilaris B, Batata M (eds) Brachytherapy oncology. New York Memorial Sloan-Kettering Cancer Center, New York, pp 83–91
131 Syed AMN, Puthawala AA, Sheikh KMA (1984) Microwave interstitial hyperthermia in the management of extensive primary and recurrent tumors. Abstracts of the 4th international symposium on hyperthermic oncology, Aarhus, Denmark, July 2–6 (D16)
132. Syed N, Puthawala AA, Sheikh KM, Rafie S (1986) Interstitial irradiation and hyperthermia in the treatment of recurrent pelvic tumors (abstr). Endocurie Hypertherm Oncol 2:220
133. Szikla G (1979) Stereotactic cerebral irradiation. Elsevier/North Holland, Amsterdam
134. Trembly BS, Richter HJ, Mechling JA (1984) The effect of antenna surface cooling on the temperature distribution of an interstitial microwave antenna array. Abstracts of the 4th international symposium on hyperthermic oncology, Aarhus, Denmark, July 2–6 (D7)
135. Trembly BS, Strohbehn TW, de Sieyes D, Douple EB (1982) Hyperthermia induction by an array of invasive microwave antennas. NCI Monogr 61:497–499
136. Visser AG, Martina HJ, Van Rhoon GC (1984) RF interstitial hyperthermia: phantom measurements and computer simulations for different needle configurations. Abstracts of the 4th international symposium on hyperthermic oncology, Aarhus, Denmark, July 2–6 (D1)
137. Visser AG, Van Rhoon GC, Hoogenboom J, De RU V, Levendag PC (1987) An interstitial hyperthermia system at 27 MHz. Int J Hyperthermia 3:598
138. Vora N, Forell B, Joseph C, Lipsett J, Archambeau JO (1982) Interstitial implant with interstitial hyperthermia. Cancer 50:2518–2523
139. Vora N, Luk KH, Forell B, Lipsett JA, Findley D, Desai K, Penzer R, Covel J, Wong JYC (1986) Interstitial LCF hyperthermia for advanced cancers of the cervix (abstr). Endocurie Hypertherm Oncol 2:221
140. Wait JR (1985) Comments on ferromagnetic implants in hyperthermia. IEEE Trans Biomed Eng 32:707–708
141. Weller SA, Goffinet DR, Goode RL, Bagshaw MA (1976) Carcinoma of the oropharynx, results of megavoltage radiation therapy in 305 patients. AJR 126:236–247
142. Wong TZ, Strohbehn JW, Smith KF, Trembly BS, Douple EB, Coughlin CT (1984) An interstitial microwave antenna array system (IMAAH) for local hyperthermia. Abstracts of the 4th international symposium on hyperthermic oncology, Aarhus, Denmark, July 2–6 (D9)
143. Yabumoto E, Suyama S (1984) Interstitial radiofrequency hyperthermia in combination with external beam radiotherapy. In: Overgaard J (ed) Hyperthermic oncology 1984, vol 1. Taylor and Francis, London, pp 579–582
144. Yerushalmi A, Jaffe D, Weber R (1986) Thermocouple thermometry in RF fields (abstr). Proceedings of VIIIth meeting of hyperthermic oncology (ESHO), Tiberias, Israel, Sept 22–25, pp 28–29

2 Hyperthermia in Urology

K.-H. BICHLER, W. L. STROHMAIER, J. STEIMANN, and S. H. FLÜCHTER

2.1 Introduction

Presently hyperthermia in urology is mainly used in the treatment of bladder and prostatic cancer. Additionally local hyperthermia is in use in the treatment of benign prostatic hyperplasia (BPH) and chronic abacterial prostatitis. Several groups are now investigating the effect of local hyperthermia on the bladder wall as well as on the prostate. Equipment is to hand which makes clinical testing possible.

There are still many unanswered questions regarding the use of hyperthermia, e.g., concerning the duration and intensity of the hyperthermia treatment, the number of treatments, and the combination of hyperthermia with other methods such as surgery, radiation, and chemotherapy. When combining hyperthermia with other treatments, there is also the question of the timing of the hyperthermia – whether is should be applied with chemotherapy simultaneously , or whether chemotherapy should precede or folow hyperthermia. These questions are of clinical relevance and are being investigated at present.

While hyperthermia in the treatment of bladder and prostatic cancer is being investigated clinically, there are not yet any experimental or clinical designs for using hyperthermia in renal cancer or in tumors of the testes and penis. Renal tumors in particular, which are located deep in the tissue, can, like deep-seated tumors in general, hardly be accessed by hyperthermia because of technical difficulties [15].

For anatomical reasons, however, hyperthermia of the bladder has much to recommend it since the urothelium of the bladder is a retroceded surface. Thus hyperthermia of a bladder tumor is a treatment of the surface of a "superficially" located tumor. There is a similar situation with the prostate, which can be accessed transrectally so that hyperthermia of the surface is rendered possible. One must not forget, however, that special hyperthermia equipment has to be used for the areas in question. In the following we shall report on the possibilities of treatment in the bladder and the prostate.

2.2 Hyperthermia of the Urinary Bladder

2.2.1 Development of the Use of Hyperthermia in Bladder Cancer

The investigations thus far performed on local hyperthermia of the bladder have made use of arterial perfusion, water baths, body cavity perfusion, ultrasound, or microwaves or alternating currents of different wavelengths to produce therapeutically effective temperatures. Initially warm water flow had been used for local hyperthermia of the bladder.

Most of the papers published on local hyperthermia of the bladder have dealt with hyperthermic perfusion of the bladder lumen [10, 12, 21, 22, 26, 27]. The technical procedure is as follows: a bladder rinsing liquid at a set temperature is perfused into the bladder via a roller pump. Temperature measurements are taken at the entry and the exit of the rinsing liquid. Criticism of the papers has mainly related to the fact that exact experimental investigations on the model tumors were not made. Moreover clinical results can only be judged with qualifications since there are considerable differences in staging, control criteria, and control periods. As far as can be ascertained local hyperthermia of the bladder as monotherapy for bladder cancer results in complete remission in 13%–20% of cases and in partial remission in 51%–83%. One essential point of criticism with this regimen is the fact that the circulation of rinsing liquid produces therapeutic temperatures of about 43 °C only at the surface of parts of the bladder wall. Our own investigations with tumor-bearing and non-tumor-bearing bladders in dogs demonstrated that hyperthermic perfusion does not produce therapeutically effective temperatures in the deeper layers of the bladder wall [2, 13]. Due to a reactive dilatation of the vessels there is such a quick removal of heat that with homogeneous distribution of temperature in the different areas of the bladder wall there might be the

Table 2.1. Transurethral hyperthermia: technical data

Frequence	300 – 500 kHz
Wavelength	1000 m
Max. effort	250 W
Filling medium	0.17% NaCl
Electric conductivity of bladder wall	3.5 m S/cm
Bladder temperature	43 °C

danger of a subtherapeutic rise in temperature in the deeper layers of the tumor, which might cause tumor progression.

For these reasons our own investigations were aimed at developing a technique to replace hyperthermic perfusion and guarantee homogeneous heating of the bladder wall at therapeutically effective temperatures. Preliminary results on animals demonstrated that high frequency current of adequate wavelength was appropriate to heat the bladder wall homogeneously and could thus be used to replace perfusion, which as stated above, produces superficial inhomogeneous heating only. An initial experimental investigation on an anatomical model of the pelvic cavity demonstrated that high frequency alternating current of long wave range (500 kHz, 1000 m wavelength) (with a maximum functional capacity achieved at 250 W) and a bladder filling medium of a specific electric conductivity of 3.5 S/cm presented the best therapeutic preconditions. A 0.17% sodium chloride solution was the approach to fulfil most closely the demand of an ideal current quality as well as an ideal bladder filling medium [13] (Table 2.1). With the supposition of a ball-like configuration of the bladder, almost homogeneous heating of the bladder can be achieved. Our hyperthermia equipment was developed on the basis of these data. The source of heat now is a modified 24 Charr endoscope (Fig. 2.1). The tip of the endoscope serves as an active inner electrode, while conventional coagulation electrodes, which are tied to the epigastrium, serve as inactive outer electrodes. To avoid side-effects of hyperthermia on the urethra and on the bladder the shaft and the tip of the instrument are teflonized. Thermocouples placed endoscopically allow homogeneous temperature measurement in all parts of the bladder (Fig. 2.2). The temperatures generated by the high frequency generator are regis-

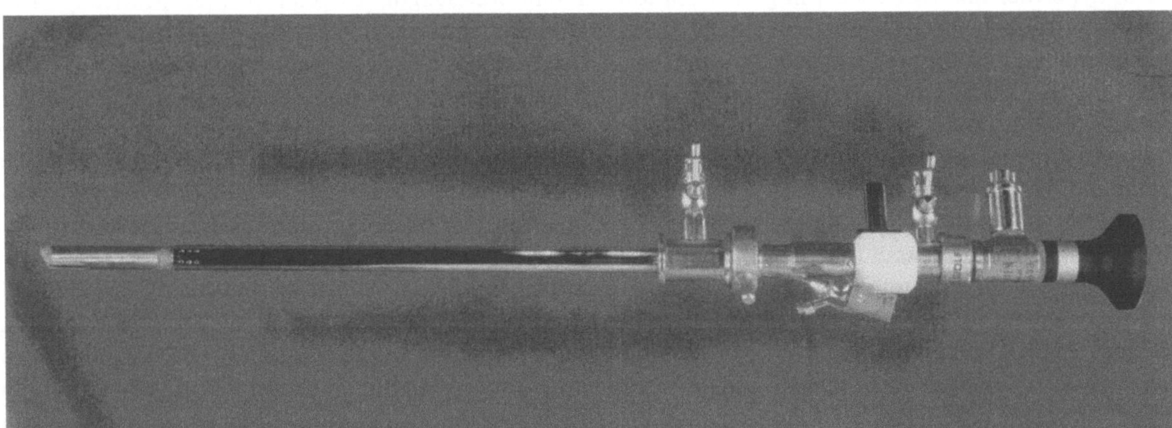

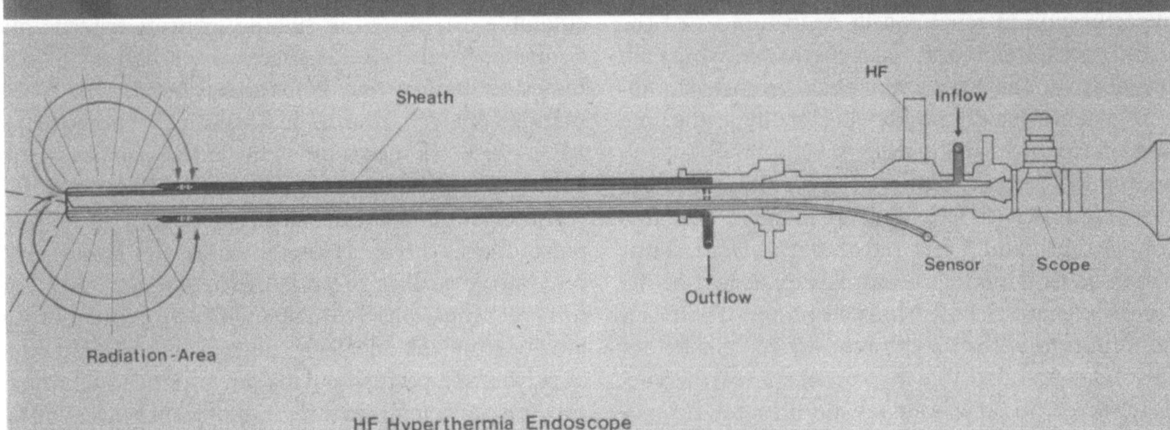

Fig. 2.1. Endoscope used for transurethral high frequency hyperthermia (Wolf, Knittlingen, W. Germany)

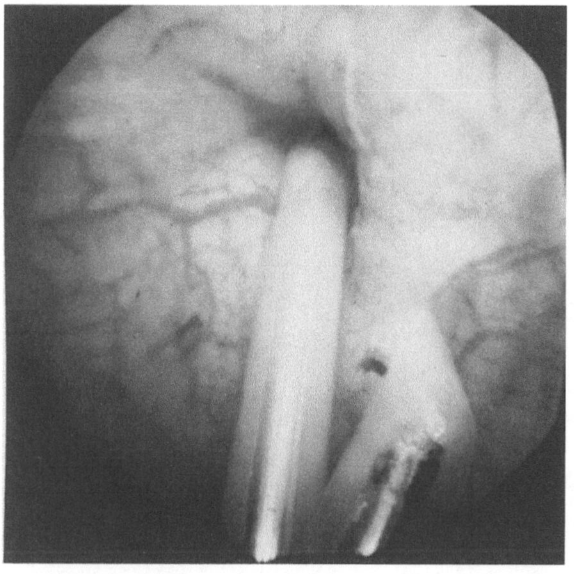

Fig. 2.2. Thermocouples being placed into the bladder wall under endoscopic control

tered and supervised. To avoid heat accumulation close to the high frequency radiation zone, rinsing liquid is circulated by means of a roller pump and by heat exchangers (Fig. 2.3).

2.2.2 Animal Experiments on Hyperthermia of the Bladder

With the instrument developed in our department, experimental trials on dog bladders as well as on Brown-Pearce carcinomas of rabbits were carried out [2, 13, 14]. In artificially induced bladder carcinomas (G_3), we found that exposure to caused 43 °C on 3 consecutive days for 60 min each time caused necrotic tissues as early sequelae in the tumors, in contrast to the tumors which had not been treated in this way. Macroscopically we found considerably reduced tumor volumes as late sequelae after 3 weeks. Histologically extended tumor necroses could be seen, though none of them was complete. The main side-effect was transitory damage of unaffected tissue adjacent to the tumor, involving vesiculation and ballooning of the urothelium or the suburothelial structures. On the whole we saw that undifferentiated G_3 tumors of bladders of dogs responded much better to local hyperthermia than did G_1 tumors, which, like unaffected tissue, showed mainly transitory alterations. Due to the results obtained, we started using hyperthermia as monotherapy in human bladder cancer, with the intention of achieving palliation.

2.2.3 Hyperthermia as Monotherapy in Bladder Cancer

Hyperthermia alone can destroy a bladder tumor. This was demonstrated by the case of a patient suffering from transitional cell carcinoma. Immediately after hyperthermia has been started, superficial tumor necrosis was found. Macroscopically one could see damage of the tumor 1 week later. Three weeks later the tumor had disappeared completely (Fig. 2.4). In the follow-up period there were no indications of recurrence [4].

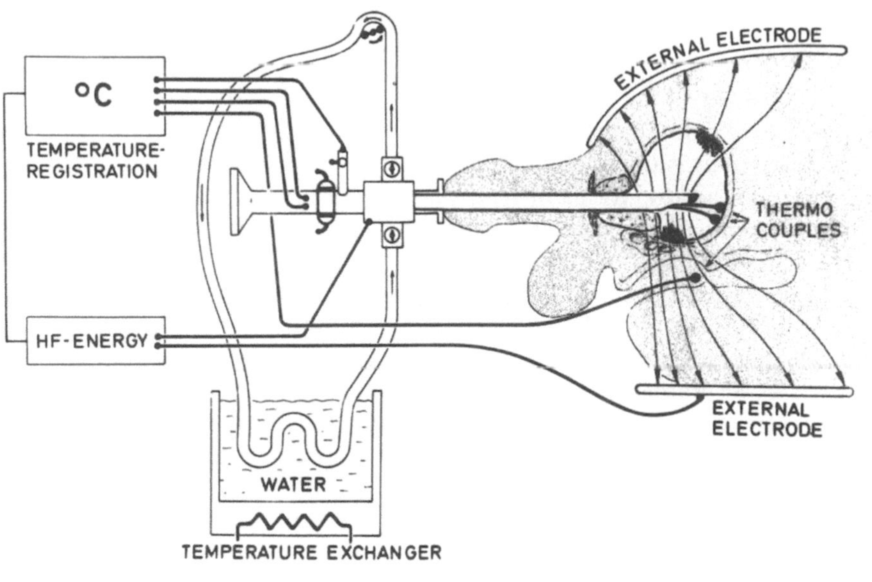

Fig. 2.3 Equipment for transurethral high frequency hyperthermia of the bladder

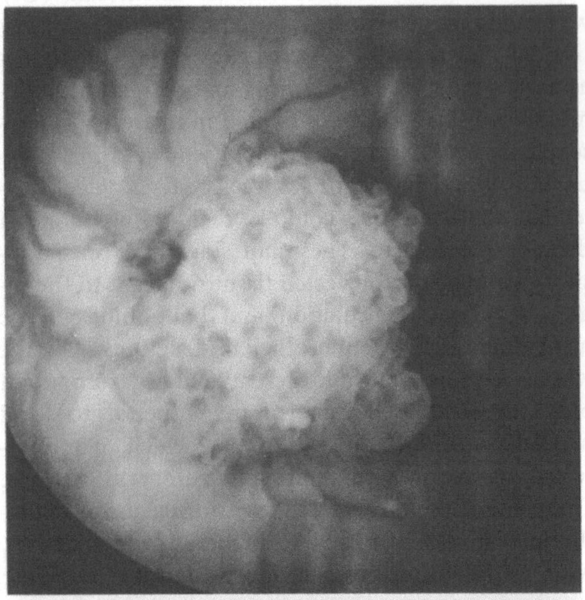
a

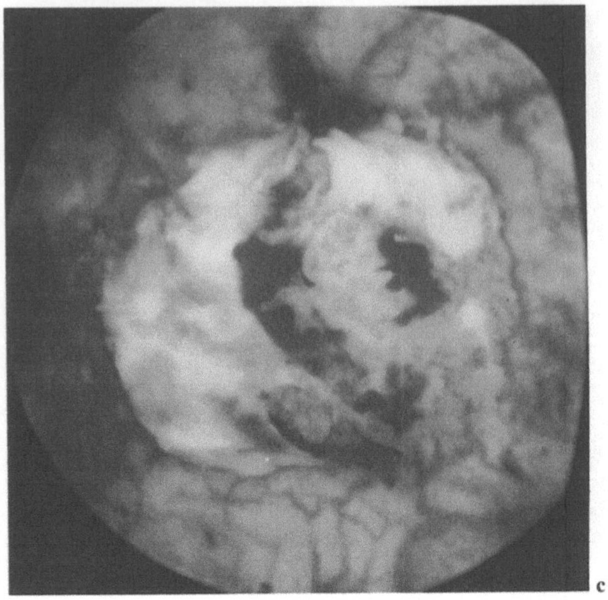
c

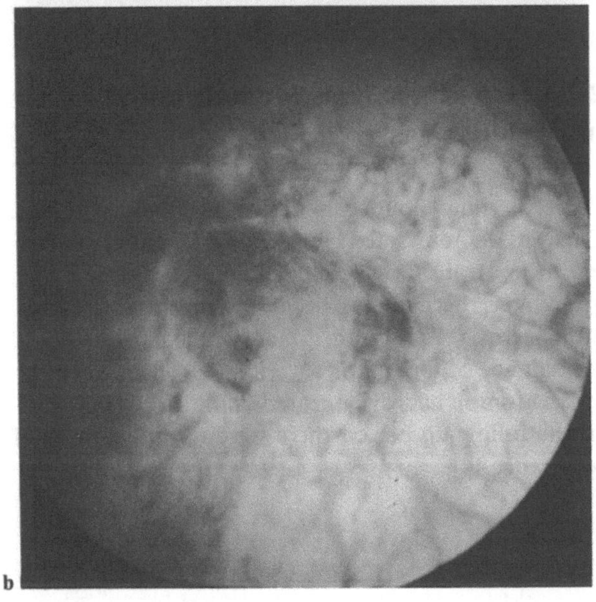
b

Fig. 2.4. a Urothelial cancer before hyperthermia (B.E. 57 year old female). **b** Effects of treatment after 1 week. **c** Complete remission of the tumor 3 weeks after hyperthermia

Fifty-nine patients (56 male, 3 female) with repeatedly pretreated (transurethral resection, partial bladder resection, cryotherapy, formalin treatment, radiation) bladder carcinomas were entered in the clinical trial; more than 90% had T_2–T_4 tumors which were poorly differentiated. The majority of patients (96%) had carcinomas of the urothelium. The others had either epitheliomas, adenocarcinomas, bladder sarcomas, or metastases of urothelial carcinomas of the renal pelvis. Similar to the results of salvage cystectomy, the 5-years survival rate among these patients tollated 19%. The essential results of our clinical trial were the observation of reduced tumor volumes, of interruption of hemorrhages, and of absence of tumors after transurethral resection in 17%; similar results were obtained in 7 out of 12 patients who had undergone cystectomy after hyperthermia. Histologically we found as early sequelae group cell necroses; 7 days after local hyperthermia there were subtotal tumor necroses and later on, stroma hyalinosis (Fig. 2.5). This hyalinosis, we think, represents fibrous tissue replacement of carcinoma tissue; such replacement did not affect the whole tumor, though. On the contrary, remainders of vital tumor tissue were found near the vessels, that is in euoxic tumor areas. The effect of hyperthermia on non-tumor-bearing tissue was a reversible bullous change of the transitional urothelium (Fig. 2.6).

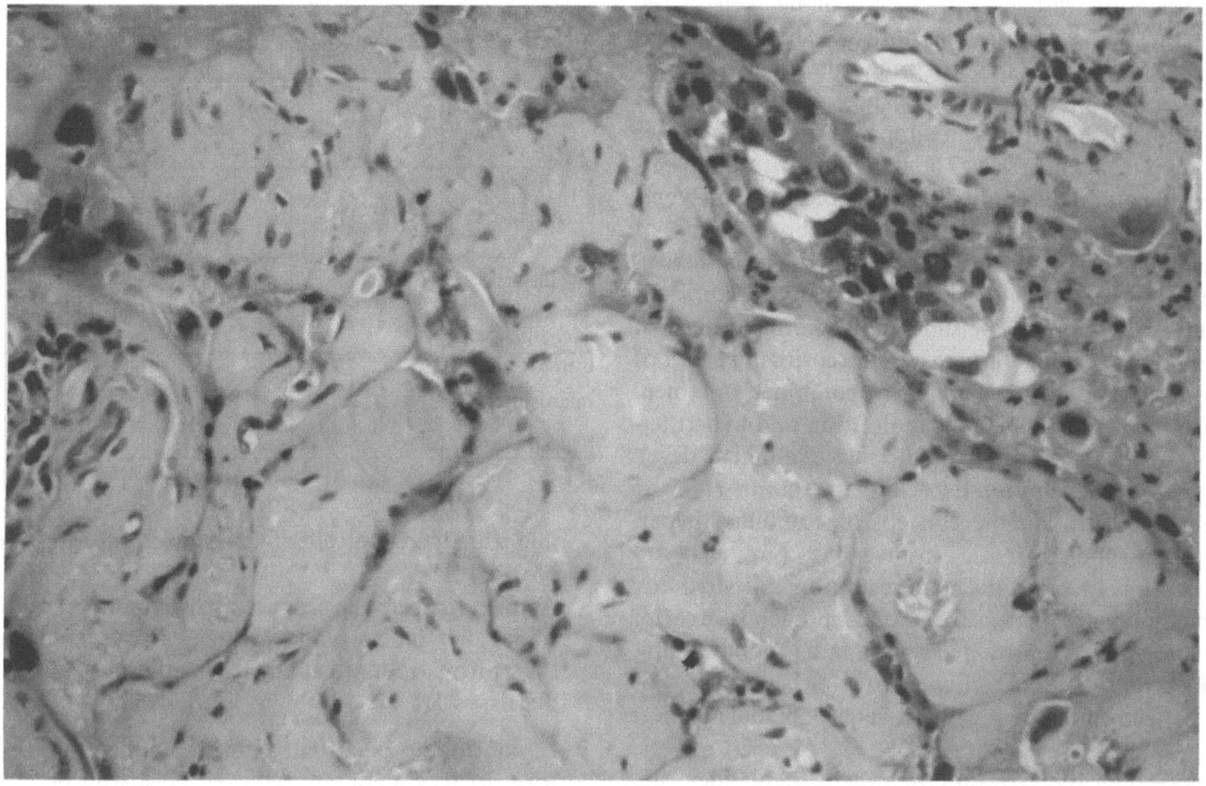

Fig. 2.5. Histological findings 3 weeks after hyperthermia of the cancer bearing human bladder: Extended stroma hyalinosis with rests of vital tumor tissue were found. H & E, ×400

2.2.4 Hyperthermia as Part of an Integrated Combined Treatment in Bladder Cancer

The results obtained in these investigations indicate that local transurethral high frequency hyperthermia has more than palliative effects on tumor tissue, particularly in the case of poorly differentiated tumors. However, hyperthermia as monotherapy does not seem suitable for curative use for bladder cancer. Because of these results we decided to apply transurethral high frequency hyperthermia as part of an integrated therapeutic concept for the treatment of bladder cancer. According to the principles of neoadjuvant therapy, as for instance described by Jakse and Frommhold in respect of the combination of radiation and cytostatics [16], we combined transurethral high frequency hyperthermia with locoregional intraarterial cytostatic microsphere infusion [11]. Radiation and most of the cytostatics that are effective in euoxic tumors and hardly show any damaging effects on anoxic cancer tissue can, be combined well with hyperthermia. The advantage of a combination with hyperthermia is the synergistic cancer cell-killing activity. Another important point of interest for the

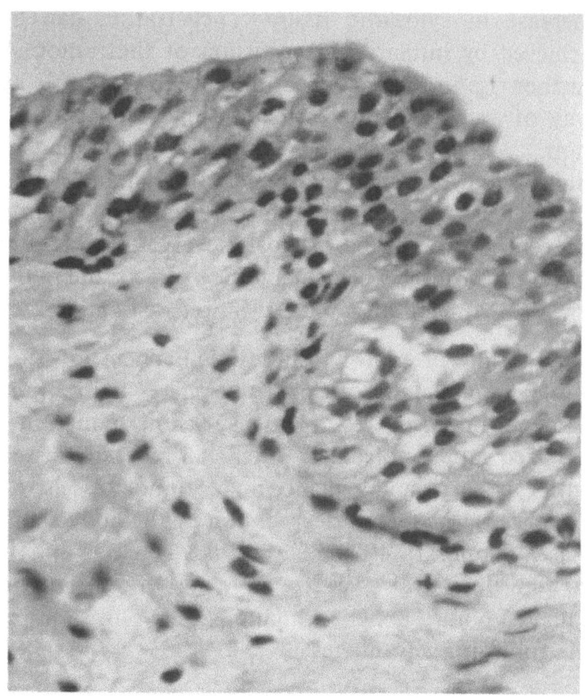

Fig. 2.6. Tissue not bearing tumor, showing reversible bullous changes of the urothelium after hyperthermia. H & E, ×300

combination with hyperthermia can be seen in the fact that euoxic tumor areas have a special thermosensitivity and thus hyperthermia alone has a cancer-damaging effect, in this cancer tissue, too – as could be demonstrated in animal and clinical studies in our department [3]. The combined use of hyperthermia and radiation leads to superadditive or synergistic cell-damaging activity when both forms of treatment are applied simultaneously. The effectiveness of radiation is increased by means of concomitant hyperthermia. The superadditive effectiveness of radiation is gained through a radiosensitizing effect of hyperthermia [35]. We prefer the combined treatment with locoregional chemoembolization and hyperthermia by means of the hyperthermia equipment developed for that purpose. Especially for tumors showing deeper infiltration the concept of combined hyperthermia and systemic intravenous but also intraarterial locoregional administration of cytostatics opens up a new perspective. This approach is superior to the application of hyperthermia as monotherapy. The promise of this combined therapy is illustrated by its effectiveness in locally advanced bladder cancer [7].

Concerning the cytostatic treatment of bladder cancer, a correlation is seen between cytostatic tissue concentration, drug efficiency, and systemic toxicity. Often when performing intravenous administration of cytostatics, the high concentration of the drug needed for treatment gives rise to systemic toxic effects. An increase in cytostatic tissue concentration can be achieved by intraarterial perfusion of the tumor. A further rise in tissue concentration seems possible by way of an intraarterial cytostatic microsphere infusion. We think that a technique combining intraarterial cytostatic microsphere infusion and hyperthermia produces, apart from the highest local drug concentration, the best cytostatic effectiveness and has the lowest rates of systemic side-effects due to the lowest peripheral drug concentration [11] (Table 2.2).

Table 2.2. Cytostatics in bladder cancer

Method	Tumorconcentration	Efficiency	Systemic toxicity
Intravenous	↑	↑	↑
Intraarterial	↑↑	↑↑	↑
Intraarterial + microspheres	↑↑↑↑	↑↑↑↑	↑
Intraarterial + microspheres + hyperthermia	↑↑↑↑	↑↑↑↑	↑

For the intraarterial cytostatic microsphere infusion (CMI) we make use of Spherex. Spherex is the trade name for microspheres. It is a suspension of micrometer sized starch molecules, which can by easily mixed with cytostatics and which occludes tumor vessels. As there is a spontaneous degradation by the body's amylase, temporary ischemia results. The half-life is 20 min.

This temporary Spherex carcinoma embolization has the following advantages:

1. Direct drug injection into cancer tissue
2. Cytostatic accumulation in cancer tissue on the one hand, with diminished systematic toxic effects due to reduced peripheral cytostatic concentration on the other
3. As demonstrated in respect of liver tumors, additional damage to bladder cancer tissue owing to the Spherex-induced tumor ischemia must also be discussed [1]

In contrast to persistent tumor embolization, this form of treatment can be used repeatedly [9]. We perform this combined treatment in case of

1. Locoregional cancer (primarily nonoperable), with the intention of obtaining tumor debulking or complete destruction so that subsequent curative operation becomes possible
2. Advanced metastasizing tumor with the purpose of achieving palliation of locally circumscribed symptomatic metastases.

The technical approach to intraarterial tumor infusion is a follows: According to the Seldinger technique, a catheter is placed through the femoral artery into the internal iliac artery and inserted downstream of the origin of the superior gluteal artery. From this position the bladder wall, including the cancer areas, can be infused via the vesical arteries (Fig. 2.7). One course of treatment consists of an infusion of 10 mg mitomycin C or 50 mg cisplatin mixed with 15 ml, i.e., 900 mg Spherex.

There is controversy as to the timing of hyperthermia in combination with cytostatics. On the one hand the addition of cytostatics before the application of hyperthermia seems possible [6]; on the other, enhancement of cytostatic activity is also described when hyperthermia is carried out before the application of the drugs [24]. Generally an enhancement in the sense of increased effectiveness can be achieved by combining hyperthermia and cytostatics. The degree of enhancement seems to depend on the form and du-

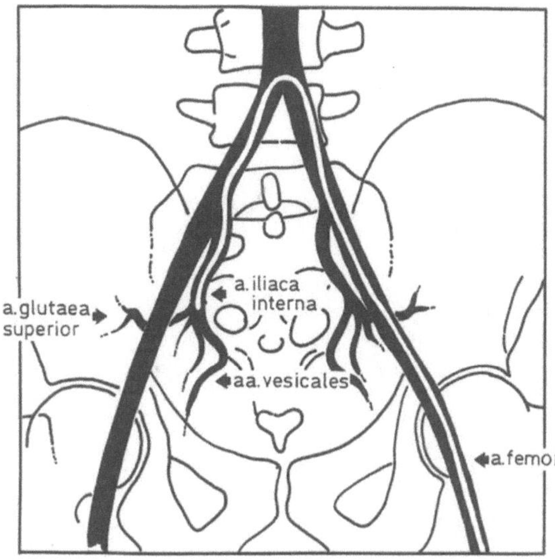

Fig. 2.7. Approach to the tumor vessels of the bladder according to the Seldinger technique

Table 2.3. Integrated therapy for bladder cancer: transurethral high frequency hyperthermia plus cytostatic microsphere infusion

	Therapy	Results
$T_{3/4}N_0M_0$ ($n = 6$) (curative, neoadjuvant)	3 MMC + hyperthermia Cystectomy ($n = 3$) TUR ($n = 3$)	CR[a]: $n = 3$; PR[a]: $n = 3$; All patients free of recurrence, 12–36 months
$T_{3/4}N_XM_X$ ($n = 6$) (palliative)	2×3 MMC + hyperthermia	*Objective findings* NC[b]: $n = 5$, 12–34 weeks; PR[a]: $n = 1$ *Subjective findings* Relief of pain; Recovery of ability to walk; Karnofski↑

MMC, mitomycin C; TUR, transurethral resection; CR, complete remission; PR, partial remission; NC, no change
[a] Histological diagnosis
[b] Autopsy: extended tumor necrosis

ration of hyperthermia, and on the single drug used in combination with hyperthermia [8]. We decided to apply hyperthermia in this series after cytostatic infusion because at this time the highest local cytostatic concentrations are seen in the carcinomas. As far as the use of hyperthermia before cytostatics is concerned, we intend to make it a future line of investigation. The application of hyperthermia and locoregional cytostatic infusions at the same time, which would be desirable because of the changes in pH, O_2 tension, and nutrient supply, apparently is not possible for technical reasons.

2.2.5 Results of Combined Hyperthermia and Locoregional Chemoembolization

Preliminary results obtained in our department in 12 patients with integrated treatment involving hyperthermia of the bladder wall and intraarterial cytostatic application with mitomycin C and a follow-up of more than 12 months will be reported (Table 2.3).

In six patients suffering from locoregional cancers, treatment was performed with a curative, neoadjuvant intention; it consisted of three courses of tumor infusion, each fallowed 24 h later by hyperthermia. One week later removal of the tumor was performed either by cystectomy or by transurethral resection of the bladder. Six patients with metastasizing tumors with local progressive metastases and complaints such as ischialgia, bone ache and inability to walk were treated by two series of three courses each at an interval of 2 weeks. The aim of treatment was palliation. The intraarterial cytostatic infusion was performed locally into the primary tumor and/or into the symptomatic metastases. Response to treatment was measured by objective criteria.

So far all patients have, after operative removal of the bladder or transurethral resection, been free of recurrence in the follow-up period of 12–36 months. Histological preparations after cystectomy demonstrated cancer areas with total tumor necrosis (Fig. 2.8). Furthermore one could see some cancer areas which had remained unaffected and some showing widespread necrotic alterations (Fig. 2.8). The histological diagnosis of partial remission was made when there was tumor damage of more than 50% of the mass, compared to the histology before integrated treatment. In the perivesical fatty tissue, arteries constricted by chronic subintimal edema were demonstrated (Fig. 2.9). These findings indicate effects of treatment not only in the wall but also in the perivesical structures. Effects of treatment in metastasizing bladder cancer stage $T_{3-4}N_xM_x$ were as follows: All patients showed an improvement of their general state of health immediately after the first intraarterial cytostatic infusion and felt alleviation or elimination of symptoms. In those patients suffering from bone metastases and restricted movement the ability to walk and move was improved. Stabilization, measured as reduced or unchanged tumor volume, persisted for 12–34 weeks in five patients. These patients finally died owing to their disease. Autopsy demonstrated

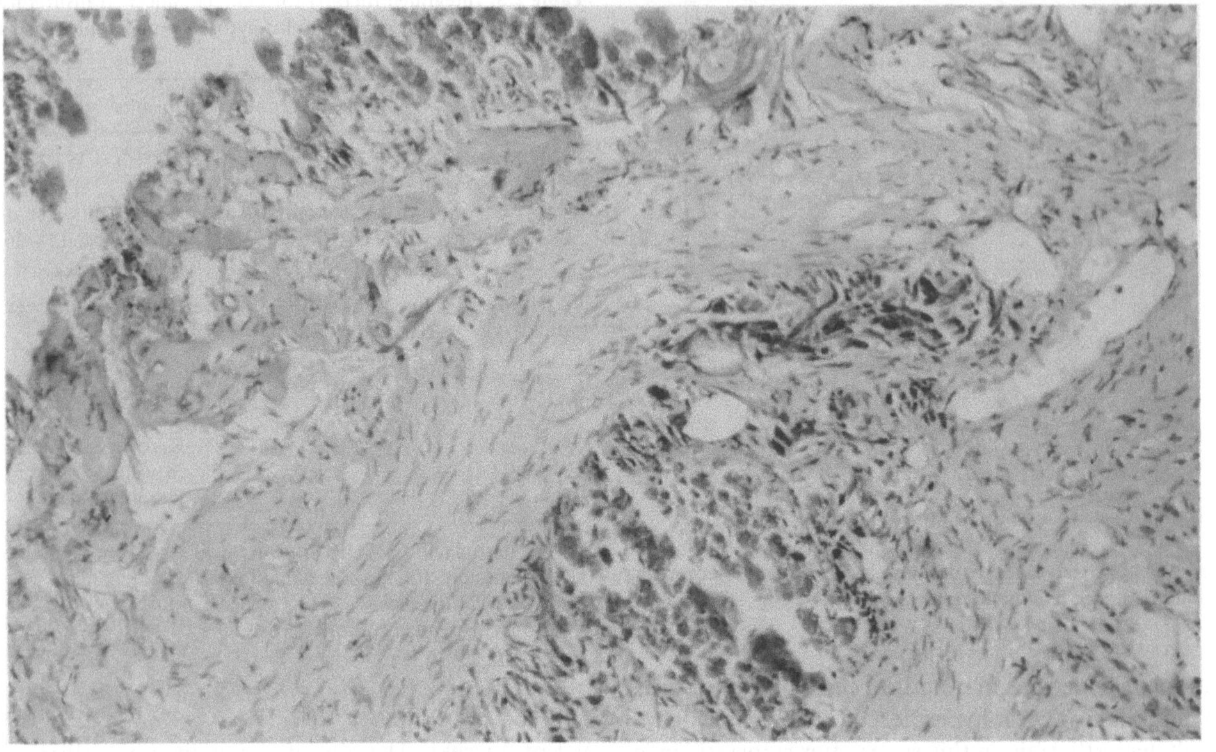

Fig. 2.8. Histological findings after combined treatment with total tumor necrosis of the bladder cancer. H & E, ×150

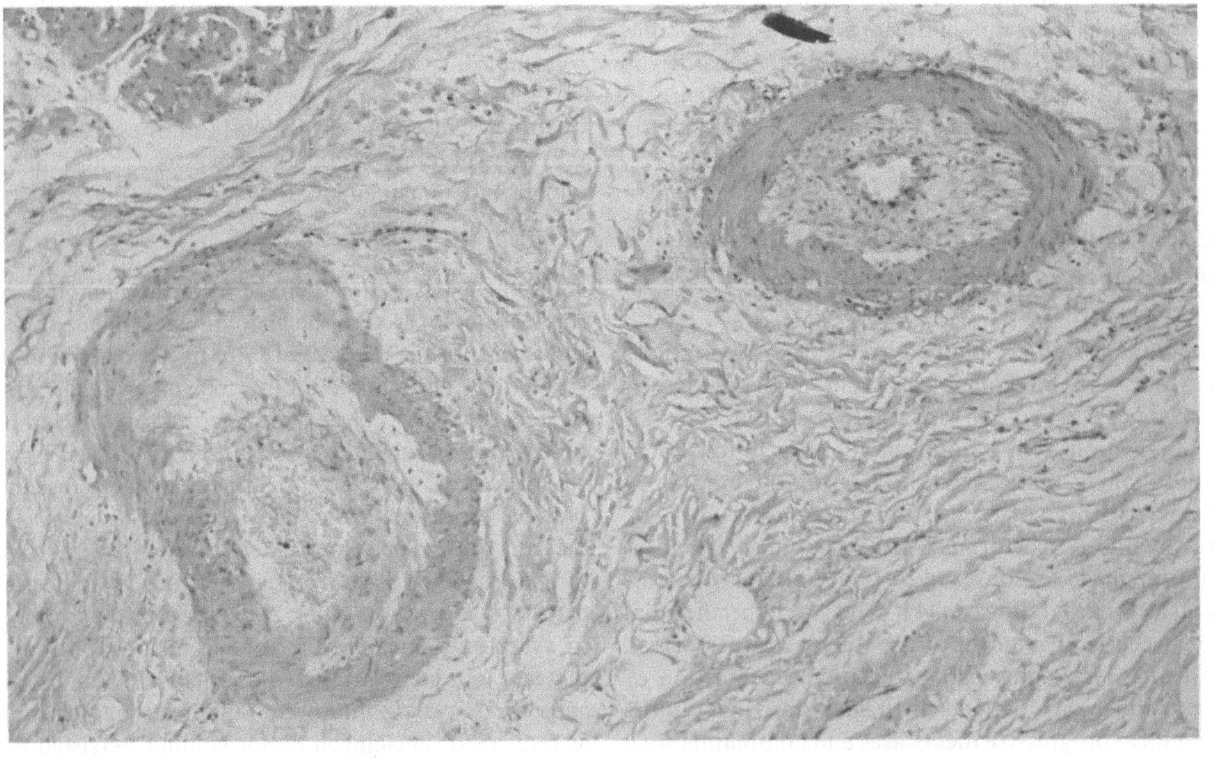

Fig. 2.9. Histological findings in the perivesical fatty tissue with considerably constricted arteries and chronic subintimal edema. H & E, ×150

vast areas of extended necrosis of the tumor. For 15 months now a patient who had impressive local tumor debulking has been free of recurrence after cystectomy and pulmonary lobectomy. Judging by the results of our animal experiments and from the experience of hyperthermia as monotherapy, we believe that combined treatment involving intraarterial microsphere infusion and transurethral high frequency hyperthermia is a method promising success for additional cancer destruction. Synergistic processes, particularly reinforcement of cytostatic effects by hyperthermia, have to be considered. The results obtained recently make us suppose that the method of treatment described above is effective as neoadjuvant therapy of locoregional (primarily inoperable) bladder cancer. It remains our hope that the survival rate for metastasizing tumors will be improved by combining hyperthermia and chemotherapy and that a decisive step towards palliation can be taken.

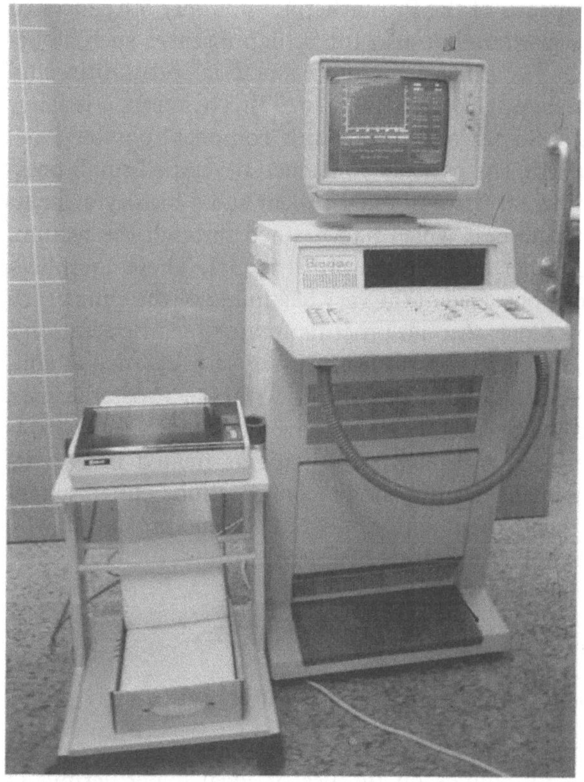

Fig. 2.10. The Prostathermer (Biodan Medical Systems, Rehovot, Israel)

2.3 Hyperthermia of the Prostate

Of particular interest is the use of hyperthermia not only in the bladder but in the prostate as well.

For a long time hyperthermia of the prostate raised a lot of difficulties because of the anatomical situation of this organ. Difficulties with thermometry prevented systematic application of hyperthermia in diseases of the prostate. In 1982 Yerushalmi et al. [40] submitted equipment for localized deep microwave hyperthermia (LDMWH, 2.45 GHz) which was used for hyperthermia treatment alone or in combination with radiotherapy or hormonal treatment in a small number of patients suffering from prostatic cancer. The follow-up results were encouraging [30].

Improved equipment for local microwave hyperthermia of the prostate was then described by Lev et al. [20] and Servadio et al. [31]. Their system made use of a water-cooled directional skirt-type antenna (915 MHz). It was demonstrated that accurate and safe hyperthermia was possible using this equipment [31].

The equipment described (Prostathermer) is available now from Biodan Medical Systems, Rehovot, Israel (Fig. 2.10). It consists of the following basic elements: A 915-MHz power source with a maximum capacity of 100 W is connected to a special applicator (a skirt-type antenna) which is introduced into the rectum and directed towards the prostate. A transurethral catheter with Luxtron fluoroptic thermometers is inserted to monitor the temperature in the prostatic urethra (Fig. 2.11). Special devices for cooling the rectal wall and for controlling temperature in the rectal wall are included. Elements for accurate placement of the applicator on the prostate are also incorporated [5, 31, 36, 37]. So far some hundred patients have been treated

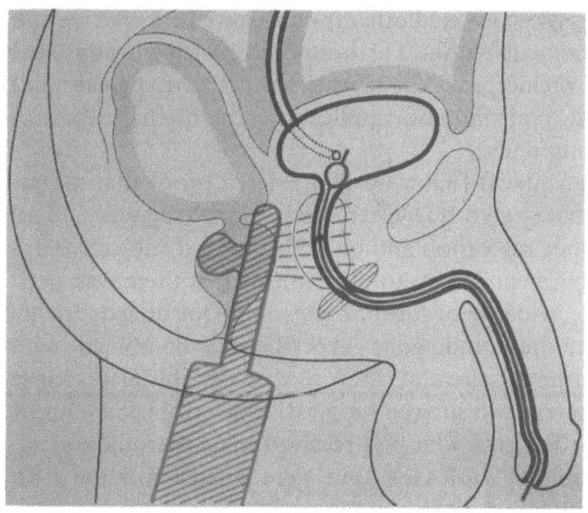

Fig. 2.11. Schematic drawing of the position of the rectal applicator of the Prostathermer directed towards the prostate

by means of the Prostathermer not only for cancer of the prostate but also for benign diseases such as benign hyperplasia, chronic abacterial prostatitis, and prostatodynia [5, 31, 32, 36, 37]. The method is fairly safe. So far only two major complications have occurred: The patients concerned developed small prostatorectal fistulas; one of them had a history of prostatic abscess which had drained through the rectum, the other had chronic proctitis [31]. These complications occurred at the very beginning of the clinical trials. Since chronic proctitis, major rectal operations, and previous prostatic abscesses were regarded as contraindications to treatment with the Prostathermer, no major complications have occurred. Our own experience with about 100 patients treated in our department has not shown complications either, except in one patient suffering from chronic prostatitis who developed urethritis after treatment.

2.3.1 Cancer of the Prostate

Several studies on the use of local hyperthermia in prostatic cancer have been performed so far. Yerushalmi et al. [40] treated a small number of patients (15) with histologically confirmed cancer of the prostate. Four had stage D disease, ten stage C disease, and one stage B disease. In five patients additional radiotherapy and in six additional hormone treatment was performed. 2.45-GHz microwave equipment with a transrectal applicator was used. Patients underwent six to nine treatments all told, of 60 min each. Intraprostatic temperature, as measured by a needle inserted into the center of the prostatic mass, was 42 °–43 °C. Radiotherapy followed hyperthermia treatment within 2 h; hormonal treatment consisted of orchiectomy (3–4 weeks prior to hyperthermia) and concomitant application of diethylstilbestrol (3 mg daily).

The clinical follow-up [30] offered proof that all patients treated by hyperthermia alone (stage B/C) had tumor regression and an objective and subjective improvement for up to 6 months. Then there was definite evidence of local progression. Out of six patients who had undergone hyperthermia combined with hormonal therapy, four showed an initial response whereas two showed progressive deterioration. Out of five patients who had received hyperthermia and radiotherapy (62 Gy), four were cured while the fifth died of his disease.

Servadio et al. [32] reported on 24 prostatic cancer patients treated with the Prostathermer (915 MHz, 42 °–43 °C). After six to ten hyperthermia sessions (once or twice weekly) shrinkage of the prostate, measured by transrectal ultrasound, was seen. Objective voiding data, e.g., urine flow rate and residual urine, could be improved, and indwelling catheters could be removed in seven out of ten patients. Symptoms such as dysuria, urgency, frequency, and pelvic discomfort improved as well. In nine patients prostatic biopsy showed downgrading or disappearance of the tumor; systematic investigations on the effect of hyperthermia on prostatic cancer tissue, however, were not performed.

Recently Szmigielski et al. [39] reported on 15 patients with advanced (T3–4NxM0–1) prostatic cancer treated by local microwave hyperthermia. The equipment used in the study consisted of a 2.45-GHz microwave source, a transrectal applicator, and miniature thermomisters YSI 400 (needle shaped) introduced into the prostatic tumor. Intraprostatic hyperthermia (43.5 °C) was maintained for 30 min. Altogether six sessions were held; treatment was subdivided into two phases of three sessions each at an interval of 4 weeks. After 6 months, 8 out of 15 patients had responded to treatment (three complete remissions, five partial remissions) as measured by ultrasound volumetry of the prostate, bone scan, alkaline phosphatase, and prostatic acid phosphatase. The main result obtained was a reduction of the volume of the prostates and, as a concomitant phenomenon, improvement of the general clinical and voiding states. In two patients bone metastases disappeared, as was documented by bone scan. As in the study conducted by Servadio et al. [32], histological effects of hyperthermia on prostatic cancer tissue were not analyzed systematically.

This was why we investigated the histological effects of microwave hyperthermia on prostatic cancer tissue [38]. Twenty patients with untreated adenocarcinomas of the prostate ($T_{1-4}N_{0-2}M_{0-1}G_{1-3}$) underwent local microwave hyperthermia with the Prostathermer prior to conventional treatment. Four hyperthermia sessions (twice weekly) of 60 min each were performed; intraprostatic temperature ranged from 42 ° to 43 °C. In order to study the effects of local microwave hyperthermia on prostatic cancer tissue, histological specimens of the prostate were taken by punch biopsy, transurethral resection, or radical prostatectomy before treatment and 1 week after the last session. The same histological effects of local microwave hyperthermia on prostatic cancer tissue could be seen in each patient. The stroma showed distinct edema and diffuse lymphoplasmacellular infiltration indicating interstitial inflammation (Figs. 2.12, and 2.13). Near the capsule, hyperemic capillary blood

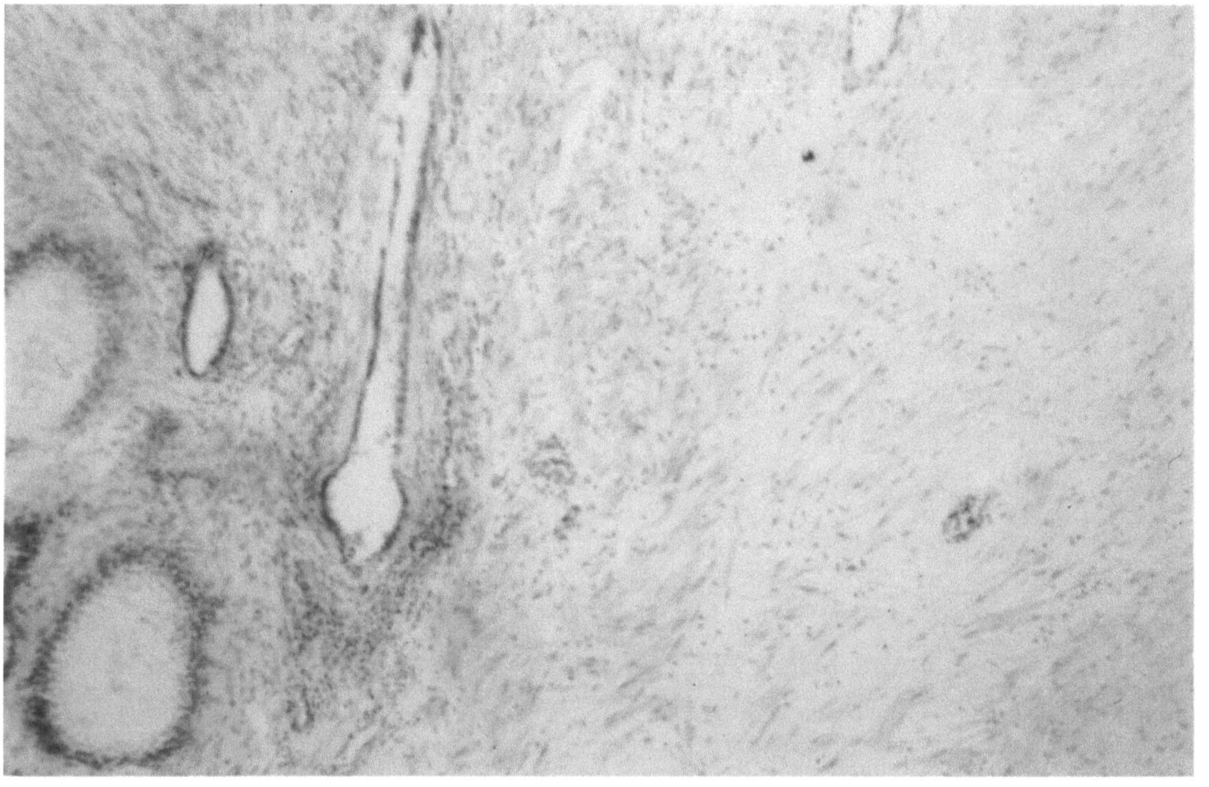

Fig. 2.12. Stromal edema after hyperthermia for prostatic cancer. H & E, ×150

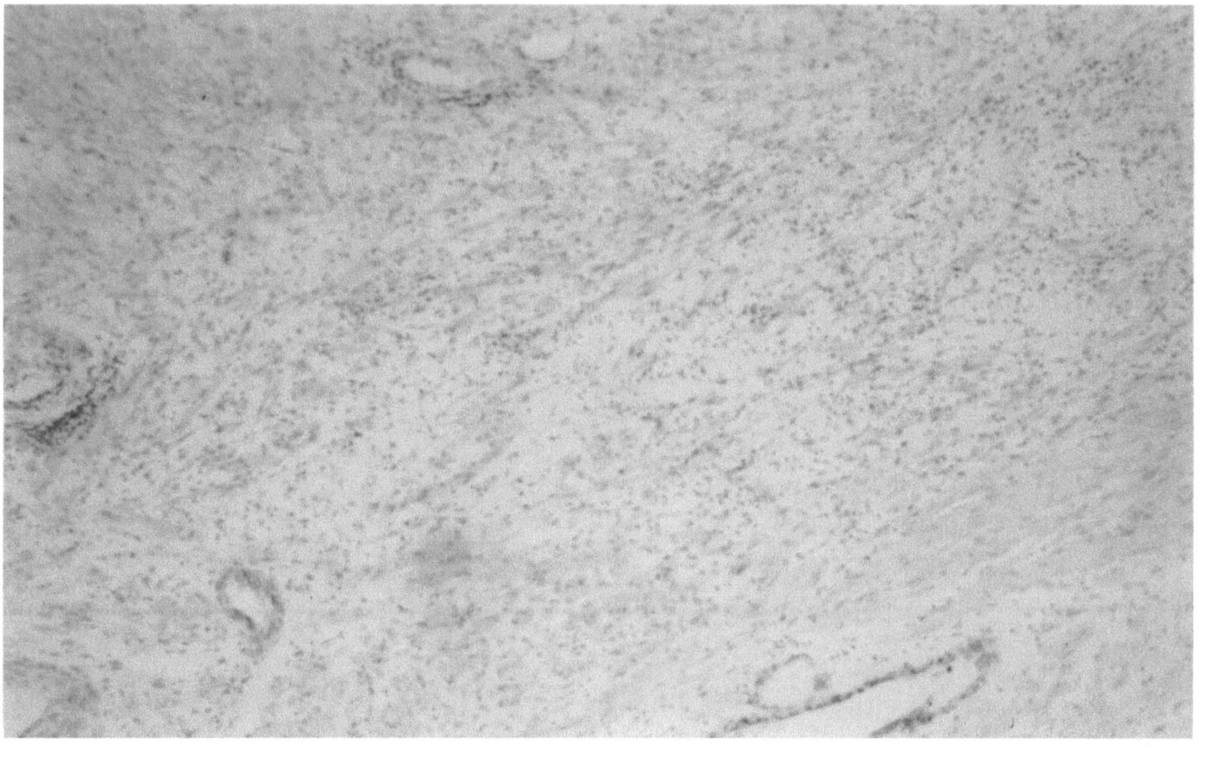

Fig. 2.13. Stromal edema with lymphoplasmacellular infiltration after hyperthermia for prostatic cancer. H & E, ×150

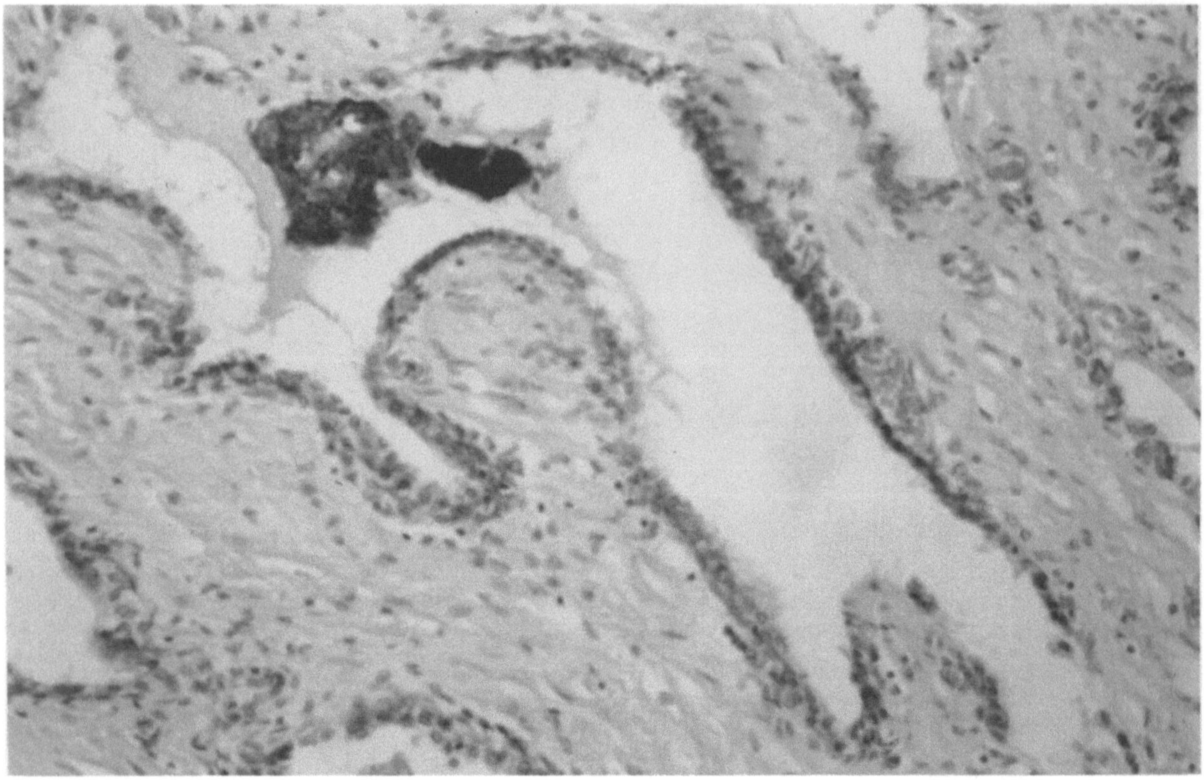

Fig. 2.14. Hyperemic capillaries with stromal hemorrhage after hyperthermia for prostatic cancer. H & E, ×200

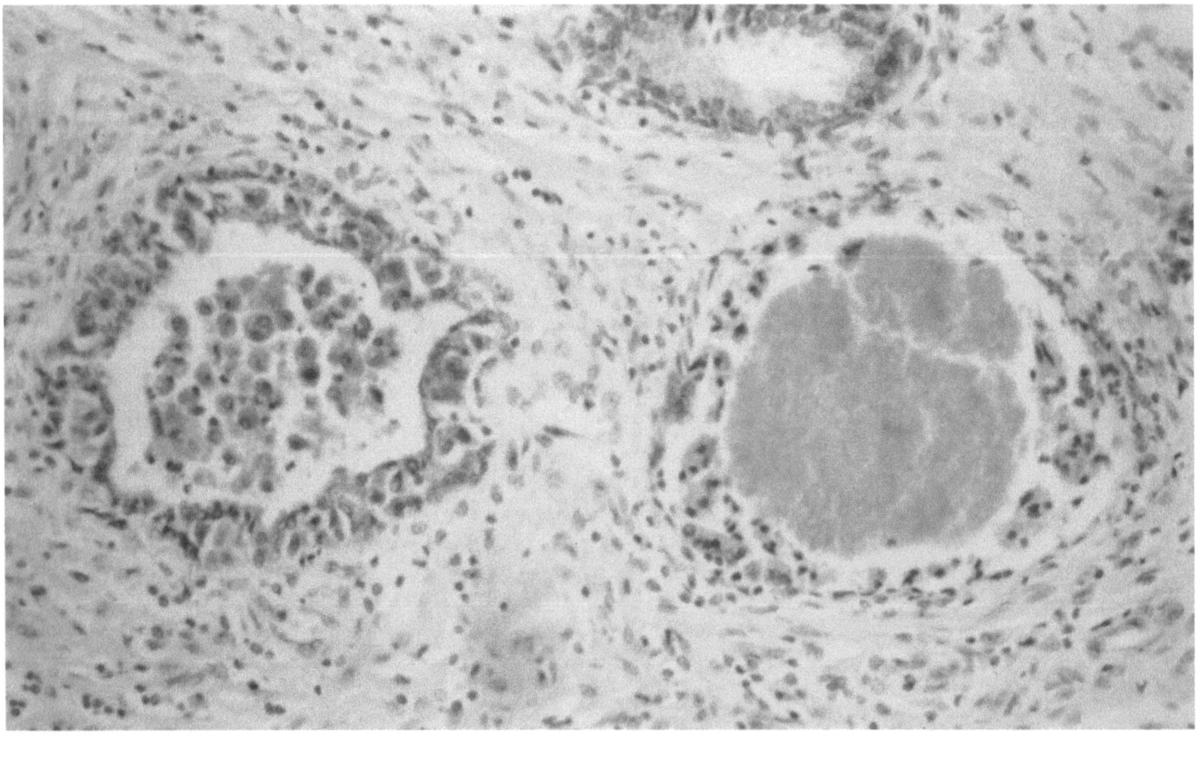

Fig. 2.15. Intraglandular macrophages laden with hemosiderin after hyperthermia for prostatic cancer. H & E, ×200

vessels with bleeding into the strome were found (Fig. 2.14). In the center of the glands macrophages laden with hemosiderin were found as a residual effect of previous bleeding (Fig. 2.15). Moreover damaged major blood vessels showed distinct swelling of the wall, and in some areas total obstruction of some vessels was ascertained. In some patients, groups of necrotic glands were found. Cytoplasm showed slight vacuolation which had, however, been found before hyperthermia, too. Evidence of tumor cell destruction by local microwave hyperthermia could not be produced in any of the patients. The histological effects on prostatic cancer tissue described here were similar to those described by Leib et al. for unaffected canine prostates [19]. Our results indicate that the shrinkage of prostatic tumors described in previous studies [32, 39] cannot be explained by histologically proben malignant cell destruction. This is supported by the fact that the shrinkage of the prostate also can be registered after hyperthermia treatment in benign prostatic diseases like BPH and chronic prostatitis [32]. Moreover it seems evident that local microwave hyperthermia should not be applied to the prostate as monotherapy in prostatic cancer. Local microwave hyperthermia might be useful as part of a combined treatment (e.g., with cytostatics, hormonal agents, or radiotherapy) as it produces distinct hyperemic alterations of the prostate. In this way the concentration of cytostatics or hormonal agents might be increased considerably. Moreover a potentiation of cytostatic action by hyperthermia treatment, found in several experimental studies [18, 25, 33, 43], has to be taken into account. Proceeding from these results we are now conducting a multicenter randomized study – in cooperation with Servadio – on the effect of combined hyperthermia and androgen deprivation on metastasizing prostatic cancer (stage D): A total of 48 patients in each center are meant to be treated according to this protocol. Three study groups are randomized. The groups are treated by buseriline or orchiectomy combined with flutamide. Group 1 receives an additional five sessions of local hyperthermia, the maximum target temperature being 42°–43°C. Group 2 receives ten hyperthermia sessions, while group 3 does not receive hyperthermia treatment. To evaluate the effects of this combined treatment the following diagnostic procedures are performed before and 6 months after hyperthermia treatment: medical check-up, prostatic acid phosphate, prostatic specific antigen, uroflowmetry, residual urine, transrectal ultrasound of the prostate, intravenous pyelography, chest X-ray, bone scan, abdominal CT scan, and prostate biopsy (aspiration and punch). The results of this study have not yet been submitted.

2.3.2 Benign Hyperplasia of the Prostate

As local microwave hyperthermia had effected a reduction of the volume of the prostate in prostatic cancer patients it seemed an obvious step to examine the effects of hyperthermia on the enlarged benign prostate as well. BPH is one of the most common diseases in elderly men causing voiding dysfunction and urinary retention. The standard treatment of BPH is surgical intervention, i.e., transurethral resection or open surgery (transvesical or retropubic prostatectomy). So far no effective noninvasive treatment is available.

Servadio et al. [32] reported on 29 patients suffering from BPH who had undergone local microwave hyperthermia treatment. Six to ten hyperthermia sessions had been held (once or twice weekly for 60 min) by means of the Prostathermer. Six months after treatment the size of the prostate had declined, and urinary flow rate and residual urine had improved. In 8 out of 13 patients it had been possible to remove the indwelling catheter. Personal complaints like frequency, urgency, nocturia, dysuria, and full bladder sensation had improved. In 1985 Yerushalmi et al. [41] reported on 29 patients suffering from BPH who had been treated by local deep microwave hyperthermia of 2.45 GHz at 43 °C. The same equipment as described above had been used [40]. The patients enrolled in the study underwent 12–15 hyperthermia sessions (twice weekly). Subjective and objective response in micturition was found. In 8 out of 11 patients indwelling catheters could be removed. Residual urine ranged from 0 to 60 ml. The maximum follow-up was 18 months.

In 1988 Yerushalmi [42] reported on 67 patients suffering from BPH who were treated according to the same scheme. Altogether 84% of 47 patients who were evaluated had improved symptoms and objective voiding signs. In the follow-up period of up to 56 months, relief from prostatic symptoms persisted in 81% of the patients. Of the indwelling catheters, 75% could be removed. Response to treatment persisted in 70% after 51 months. To corroborate the findings of these pilot studies, a multicenter study on the effects of local microwave hyperthermia on BPH in a large number of patients is currently being conducted in Israel. Preliminary results have demonstrated that local microwave hyperthermia in combination with cyproterone acetate has produced the desired effect in 75% of the BPH patients, whose indwelling catheters could be removed. Success has persisted for 1 year (personal communication Dr. Lev). Long-term results are not yet available. It is important that the success rate was not as high as in patients who had not received cyproterone acetate concomitantly, since cyproterone acetate is an antiandrogen drug that causes problems particularly in sexually active men. Final results of this study will have to be awaited before we can determine the value of hyperthermia in BPH.

2.3.3 Chronic Prostatitis and Prostatodynia

It is rather difficult to treat abacterial prostatitis and prostatodynia. Even with sufficient antibiotic treatment in mycoplasm-induced prostatitis, improvement of personal symptoms could be achieved in only 15% of patients [29]. Therapy with α-blockers and baclofen improved the urinary flow rate; the personal symptoms, however, remained uninfluenced [17, 28, 34].
The application of heat had already been recommended in the past, but no equipment had been available to heat the prostate selectively. The development of appropriate equipment for hyperthermia treatment of the prostate permitted its use in patients suffering from chronic prostatitis and prostatodynia.
Servadio et al. [32] reported on 21 patients with chronic abacterial prostatitis who had a long clinical history and had not responded to any conventional treatment. Six to ten hyperthermia sessions were held using the Prostathermer. To evaluate the effect of hyperthermia in this disease, which is beyond objective judgment, a questionnaire on the major complaints (voiding dysfunction, discomfort, pain) was used. Subjective symptoms could be improved considerably.
To test the efficacy of microwave hyperthermia in chronic abacterial prostatitis and prostatodynia we started a randomized prospective study about a year ago. A total of 96 patients with a long-standing history (of more than 12 months) of chronic abacterial prostatitis and prostatodynia (classified according to Meares [23]) have been enrolled. The following preliminary examinations have been conducted: case history, medical check-up, residual urine measurement, transrectal ultrasound of the prostate, and anoscopy. To evaluate the personal complaints, the patients have to fill in a questionnaire on urgency, frequency, dysuria, discomfort, erection, and ejaculation. The answers given are scored. Only patients with a bad score (≤ 95) are enrolled. There are 16 treatment subgroups differing along the following parameters: medication, doxycycline or placebo), temperature (39.5° or 43.0°C), treatments by the week (one or two), and duration of treatment (2 or 4 weeks). For hyperthermia treatment the Prostathermer is used.

Table 2.4. Effect of local microwave hyperthermia on chronic abacterial prostatitis and prostatodynia, as judged by the questionnaire on personal complaints

Score		$(\bar{x} \pm s)$
Before treatment	($n = 25$)	75.6 ± 14.8
After 1 week	($n = 25$)	88.7 ± 14.7
After 1 month	($n = 22$)	87.8 ± 16.8
After 3 months	($n = 13$)	83.8 ± 18.8
After 6 months	($n = 8$)	100.5 ± 11.7

Patients are reexamined 1 week and 1, 3, and 6 months after hyperthermia. The same parameters are evaluated as in the pretreatment phase.
So far 31 patients have been randomized, and 25 could be evaluated. As far as the objective parameters, i.e., uroflowmetry, residual volume, and microbiological examination, are concerned, no significant changes have been seen. The personal complaints, however, have been improved significantly, as can be seen by the questionnaires (Table 2.4). So far no striking differences have been found in the 16 subgroups; there is, however, a tendency toward better results in those patients who have received doxycycline as well. Side-effects have occurred in only one patient, who developed urethritis.
The preliminary results obtained demonstrate considerable improvement in subjective symptoms in chronic abacterial prostatitis and prostatodynia. Long-term results, however, are not yet available. Objective changes have not been seen; chronic abacterial prostatitis and prostatodynia, however, are diseases with few objective signs but dramatic subjective symptoms. Thus it is evident that the cure of subjective complaints is much more important. It is unlikely that the findings can be interpreted as placebo effects as all patients had a long-standing history and had been treated by several urologistis in various ways. There is no evidence on the mechanism of action: Apart from hyperemia of the prostate, immunological effects have

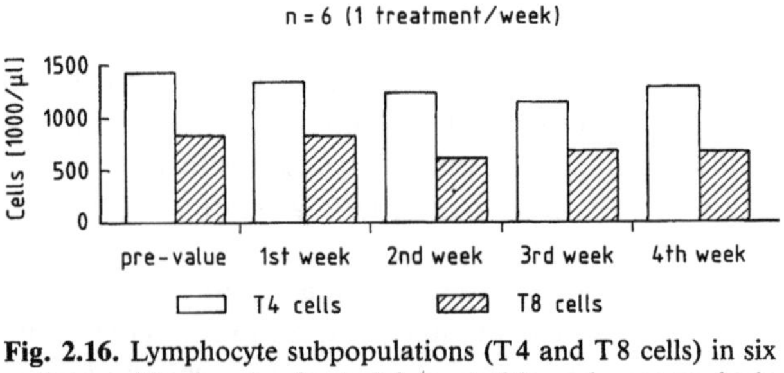

Fig. 2.16. Lymphocyte subpopulations (T4 and T8 cells) in six patients with chronic abacterial prostatitis and prostatodynia treated by microwave hyperthermia of the prostate (one treatment weekly)

to be considered. In six patients who had been examined on parameters of the cellular immunological system, a temporary decrease in T-lymphocytes (T4 and T8 cells) was found (Fig. 2.16).

In our opinion local microwave hyperthermia is a palliative treatment modality for chronic abacterial prostatitis and prostatodynia. Most likely it is not a causal treatment. Final results of our study will have to be awaited before we can define the significance of hyperthermia in chronic prostatitis and prostatodynia.

2.4 Conclusions

Our own investigations as well as those by other groups in Israel, Poland, and Japan on the use of hyperthermia in urology have demonstrated that hyperthermia as monotherapy has no sufficient tumor-damaging effect. The inclusion of hyperthermia in an integrated tumor treatment regimen, however, seems to promise success: the combination of hyperthermia and radiation or systemic or local chemotherapy, and particularly in prostatic cancer the combination of hyperthermia and hormonal treatment, seems promising. Various investigations have shown that the effectiveness of treatment is intensified by combined treatment.

Moreover hyperthermia can be used not only in the treatment of bladder and prostatic cancer but also in benign diseases, i.e., BPH, chronic prostatitis, and prostatodynia. Preliminary results of clinical trials are promising. Long-term results will have to be awaited.

References

1. Aigner KR (1985) Regionale Chemotherapie der Leber, isolierte Perfusion, intraarterielle Infusion und Resektion. In. Eckhard S, Holzner SK, Nagel GA (eds) Contribution to oncology. Karger, Basel
2. Bichler K-H, Harzmann R (1982) Lokale Hyperthermie beim Harnblasenkarzinom. Fortschr Urol Nephrol 19:83–87
3. Bichler K-H, Harzmann R, Fastenmeier K, Flachenecker G, Altenähr E, Gericke D, Flüchter SH (1982) Ergebnisse der lokalen transurethralen Hochfrequenzhyperthermie beim Harnblasenkarzinom. Urologe [A] 21:12–19
4. Bichler K-H, Flüchter SH, Steimann J, Strohmaier WL (1989) Combination of hyperthermia and cytostatics in the treatment of bladder cancer. Urol Int 44:10–14
5. Bichler K-H, Strohmaier WL, Flüchter SH, Lev A (1988) Mikrowellenhyperthermie bei chronischer Prostatitis und Prostatopathie. Niere Blase Prostata aktuell 1:6–8
6. Bowden GT, Kasuni H, Sim D (1983) Sequence dependence for the hyperthermic potentiation of cis-diamine diechloroplatinum (II) induces cytotoxicity and DNA damage. Proc 3rd annual meeting North-Americân hyperthermia group (NAHG), 26 Feb–3 March, San Antonio, Tex, pp 161–162
7. Cant JD, Brausi M, Soloway MS (1985) Adjuvant chemotherapy for locally advanced bladder cancer. World J Urol 3:115–119
8. Dahl, O (1988) Interaction of hyperthermia and chemotherapy. In: Issels RB, Wilman W (eds) Applications of hyperthermia in the treatment of cancer. Springer, Berlin Heidelberg New York. pp 157–160
9. Davis SI, Illum L, McVie JG, Tomlinson E (1984) Microspheres and drug therapy, pharmaceutical, immunological and medical aspects. Elsevier, Amsterdam
10. England MR, Anderson JD, Minasion H, Marshall VR, Molland EA, Blandy JP (1976) The therapeutic application of hyperthermia in the bladder. Br J Urol 47:849–852
11. Flüchter SH, Bichler K-H, Laberke HG, Wilbert DM (1988) Neoadjuvant local treatment of locoregional advanced bladder cancer. Regional Cancer Treat 1:50–54
12. Hall RR, Schade ROK, Swinney J (1974) Effects of hyperthermia on bladder cancer. Br Med J 2:593–594
13. Harzmann R (1980) Hochfrequenzhyperthermie beim Harnblasenkarzinom. Monographie. Urban and Schwarzenberg, München
14. Harzmann R, Bichler K-H, Altenähr E, Flachenecker G, Fastenmaier F (1980) Experimentelle Grundlagen und klinische Ergebnisse der transurethralen lokalen Hochfrequenzhyperthermie beim Harnblasenkarzinom. Verh Dtsch Ges Urol 31:101–104
15. Howard GCW, Bleehan NH (1988) Clinical experience in the combinations of hyperthermia with chemotherapy or radiotherapy. In: Issels RB, Wilmans W (eds) Application of hyperthermia in the treatment of cancer. Springer, Berlin Heidelberg New York, pp 214–221
16. Jakse G, Fritsch E, Frommhold H (1985) Combination of chemotherapy and irradiation for non-resectable bladder carcinoma. World J Urol 3:121–123
17. Janssen PL, Kukahn R, Spieler K-H, Wiessbach W (1983) Zur Psychosomatik der chronischen Prostatitis. In: Brunner H, Krause W, Rothauge CF, Weidner W (eds) Chronische Prostatitis. Schattauer, Stuttgart, pp 261–271
18. Juvenar AS, Chitnis MO, Advani SH (1987) In vitro modulation of adriamycin and mitoxantrone cytotoxicity by hyperthermia and diazepam in human chronic myeloid leukemia cells. Neoplasma 34:199–203
19. Leib Z, Rothem A, Elv A, Servadio C (1986) Histological observations in the canine prostate treated by local microwave hyperthermia. Prostate 7:93–102
20. Lev A, Leib Z, Servadio C, Shtrikman S, Treves D (1984) Heat profiles of 915 MHz skirt-type antenna. Abstracts of IV international symposium on hyperthermic oncology, July 2–6, Aarhus, Denmark
21. Ludgate CM, McLean M, Carswall GF, Newsam JE, Pettigrey RT, Selby Tulloch W (1976) Hyperthermic perfusion of the distended urinary bladder in the management of transitional cell carcinoma. Br J Urol 47:841–848
22. Lunglmayer G, Czeck K, Eisesenhofer W, Kellner G, Zechnert F (1973) Experimentelle Untersuchungen über die Wirkung temporärer Hyperthermie auf Blasentumoren. Urol Int 28:314–321
23. Meares EM, Stamey TA (1968) Bacteriologic localization

patterns in bacterial prostatitis and urethritis. Invest Urol 5:429–518
24. Murthy MS, Khandekar JD, Travis JD, Scanon EF (1984) Combined effect of hyperthermie (HT) and platin compounds in vivo and in vitro on murine and human tumor cells. Abstracts of IV international symposium on hyperthermic oncology. July 2–6, Aarhus, Denmark, pp 429–518
25. Nagaoka S, Kawasaki S, Karino Y, Hiraki Y, Nakanishui T (1987) In vivo effect of hyperthermia on the cellular uptake of adriamycin. J Radiat Res (Tokyo) 28:262–267
26. Nemoto R, Kati T, Mori H, Sware K, Harada M (1982) Hyperthermic irradiation of urinary bladder tumors in rabbits. Tohoku J Exp Med 137:199–205
27. Newsam JE, Law HT (1982) Hyperthermic perfusion of the distended urinary bladder in the management of recurrent transitional cell carcinoma. Br J Urol 59:64–65
28. Palmtag H, Riedasch G (1983) Medikamentöse Behandlung funktioneller Blasenentleerungsstörung bei Prostatitis. In: Brunner H, Krause W, Rothauge CF, Weidner W (eds) Chronische prostatitis. Schattauer, Stuttgart, pp 61–76
29. Peeters M, Polak-Vogelzang A, Debruyne F, Van der Veen J (1983) Abakterielle Prostatitis: mikrobiologische Daten. In: Brunner H, Krause W, Rothauge CF, Weidner W (eds) Chronische prostatitis. Schattauer, Stuttgart, pp 61–76
30. Servadio C, Leib Z (1984) Hyperthermia in treatment of prostate cancer. Prostate 5:205–211
31. Servadio C, Leib Z, Lev A (1986) Further observations on the use of local hyperthermia for the treatment of diseases of the prostate in man. Eur Urol 12:38–40
32. Servadio C, Leib Z, Lev A (1987) Diseases of prostate treated by local microwave hyperthermia. Urology 30 (2):97–99
33. Shang Wang B, Lumanglas AL, Silva J, Ruszala-Mallon VM, Durr FE (1987) Effect of hyperthermia on the sensitivity of human colon carcinoma cells to mitoxantrone. Cancer Treat Rep 71 (9):831–836
34. Stamay TA (1981) Prostatitis. J R Soc Med 74:22–40
35. Streffer C, Van Breuninger D (1987) The biological basis for tumor therapy by hyperthermia and radiation. In: Streffer C (ed) Hyperthermia and the therapy of malignant tumors. Springer, Berlin Heidelberg New York, pp 24–70
36. Strohmaier WL, Bichler K-H, Kiefer M, Lev A (1988) Mikrowellenhyperthermie bei chronischer Prostatitis bzw. Prostatopathie – vorläufige Ergebnisse. Verh Dtsch Ges Urol 39:527
37. Strohmaier WL, Bichler K-H, Kiefer M, Lev A (1988) Mikrowellenhyperthermie bei chronischer Prostatitis und Prostatodynie – vorläufige Ergebnisse. Helv Chir Acta 55:301–303
38. Strohmaier WL, Bichler K-H, Flüchter SH, Wilbert DM, Böcking A, Servadio C, Lev A (1988) Histological effects of local hyperthermia in prostatic cancer. Eur Ass Urol 8th Congress, May 18–21, London
39. Szmigielski A, Zielinski H, Schwarz B, Gil J, Sobcyzynski G, Jeljaszewicz J, Pulverer G (1988) Local microwave hyperthermia in treatment of advanced prostatic adenocarcinoma. Urol Res 16:1–7
40. Yerushalmi A, Servadio C, Leib Z, Fisherlovitz Y, Rokowsky E, Stein JA (1982) Local hyperthermia for treatment of carcinoma of the prostate: a preliminary report. Prostate 3:623–630
41. Yerushalmi A, Fishelovitz D, Singer D, Reiner I, Areilly J, Abramovivic Y, Catsenelson R, Levy E, Shani A (1985) Localized deep microwave hyperthermia in the treatment of poor operative risk patients with benign prostatic hyperplasia. J Urol 133:873–876
42. Yerushalmi A (1988) Localized, non-invasive deep microwave hyperthermia for the treatment of prostatic tumors: the first 5 years. In: Issels RD, Wilmans W (eds) Application of hyperthermia in the treatment of cancer. Springer, Berlin Heidelberg New York, pp 141–146

3 Experimental and Clinical Studies of Hyperthermia for Carcinoma of the Esophagus *

K. SUGIMACHI and H. MATSUDA

3.1 Introduction

The application of hyperthermia to treat malignant tumors is not a new concept. To Hippocrates (470–377 B.C.), the "Father of Medicine", is attributed the statement that "Those who cannot be cured by medicine can be cured by surgery. Those who cannot be cured by surgery can be cured by hyperthermia. Those who cannot be cured by hyperthermia are probably incurable."

Interest in hyperthermia was revived when Dr. W. Busch treated a patient with a facial sarcoma. This lesion disappeared in the presence of erysipelas, in 1866. Since then, numerous basic studies have shown hyperthermia to be an effective modality for treating cancer. Patients with carcinoma of the esophagus are now benefiting from hyperthermia treatment. The important technical problem in such cases has been that application of heat to the esophageal lesion from the body surface is not feasible. In ongoing experiments with various designs and setups, an orally inserted radiofrequency has been developed. This method is devoid of all hazards and repeated application presents no problems.

Hyperthermia treatment alone, however, will not suffice in cases of esophageal cancer. Combined chemotherapy, irradiation, and hyperthermia has synergistic effects and the benefits are substantial for these patients.

As the long-term results in patients with esophageal cancer are the poorest among patients with malignant lesions of the alimentary tract, hyperthermia warrants attention as a possible breakthrough modality for this morbid condition. The basic research, related procedures, and results are described herein.

* Reprinted with permission from Surgery, Gynecology & Obstetrics, Journal of Surgical Research, European Surgical Research, and Journal of Surgical Oncology.

3.2 Biological Basis for Prescription of the Combination of Hyperthermia, Chemotherapy, and Irradiation

There are many experimental reports concerning the antitumor effect of hyperthermia [1, 2]. In this chapter, a few fundamental experiments are described in which it is emphasized that hyperthermia combined with chemotherapy and irradiation is more effective than chemotherapy or irradiation alone.

3.2.1 Hyperthermo-chemo-radiotherapy for Treating Ehrlich Ascites Tumor in Mice

Maximum antitumor effects and minimum side-effects have to be considered when designing treatment for carcinoma of the esophagus. In recent years, increasing attention has been devoted to hyperthermia because it enhances effects of radiation and drugs such as bleomycin [3, 4]. As radiation and chemotherapy are usually applied as combined therapy in cases of carcinoma of the esophagus, combined studies on hyperthermo-chemo-radiotherapy using laboratory animals were carried out.

DDD strain male mice were given 2×10^6 Ehrlich ascites tumor cells into the right thigh intramuscularly and 10 days later these mice were used for the experiments.

A thermostatically regulated water bath was the heat source. The ten mice on the apparatus were immersed in the water bath so that the tumors were placed approximately 1.0 cm below the water surface. The mice were left for 30 min in this 42.5°C water bath. Intravenous injection of 34 mg/kg bleomycin was given via a tail vein, the dose being 1/10 LD_{50}/mouse. X-irradiation was given with a conventional X-ray generator at a dose of 30.6 rad/min.

To clarify the effects of the combination of hyperthermia, bleomycin, and X-irradiation, the following experiment was carried out. The mice were divided into five groups – group I: hyperthermia at 42.5°C for 30 min (HTM)+1/10 LD_{50} bleomycin i.v. (BLM); group II. HTM+2 Gy X-irradiation (2R); group III: BLM+2R; group IV: HTM+BLM+2R; group V: untreated control group. Hyperthermia and irradiation were given simultaneously, and when giving chemotherapy and hyperthermia or radiotherapy in combination, bleomycin was intravenously injected just before the treatments.

The median values of the tumor growth rates at 6 weeks after inoculation were 5.7 for the control group, 3.0 for HTM+BLM, 2.3 for HTM+2R, 2.5 for BLM+2R, and finally 0.5 for the combination of all three modalities. There were statistically significant differences between the group treated with all three modalities and the three groups given a combination of only two modalities each (Table 3.1).

The survival rates at 13 weeks after inoculation were 0% for the control group, 30% for HTM+BLM, 40% for HTM+2R, 50% for BLM+2R, and 80% for HTM+BLM+2R. The highest survival rate was obtained with the combination of all three modalities.

This study confirmed that:

1. The combined administration of hyperthermia, bleomycin, and X-irradiation led to a significant antitumor effect
2. With a combination of the three modalities, simultaneous application revealed a maximal thermal enhancement with no side-effects.

In cancer therapy, the combination of hyperthermia and radiation shows great promise because these modalities act synergistically [5]. However, the interaction between hyperthermia and radiation is complex, and in general the magnitude of the thermal sensitization depends on the degree and duration of hyperthermia [6], and also on the dose given [7]. When a large dose of ionizing radiation or exposure to a high temperature over an extended period is prescribed to obtain a better tumoricidal effect, normal tissue is also damaged [8]. Therefore, to improve the therapeutic effect of combined hyperthermia–radiation treatment, the sequence and timing of the two modalities are vital [9]. Thus, in the present study, to avoid increasing the dose of irradiation and/or heat, we added one more therapeutic agent to the regimen. As a result, the combination of the three modalities, at doses which individually had no effect on the growth of the tumor, brought about a significant antitumor effect, compared with the results of any combination of two modalities. In other words, the merit of the combination of the three modalities is an enhancement of tumoricidal effects and a reduction in the side-effects of each modality, as a result of the diminished dose of each. These results show the merit of the combined effects of hyperthermia with irradiation and chemotherapy.

Table 3.1. Effects of various combinations of hyperthermia, chemotherapy, and irradiation in mice

Groups	No. of mice	Tumor growth rates	Survival (%)
I. HTM+BLM	10	3.0	30
II. HTM+2R	10	2.3	40
III. BLM+2R	10	2.5	50
IV. HTM+BLM+2R	10	0.5*	80
V. Control	10	5.7	0

* Significant differences compared with the other four groups ($P<0.05$)

3.2.2 Hyperthermo-chemo-radiotherapy and the Human Esophageal Squamous Cell Line KSE-1

It has been reported that hyperthermia alone is not lethal to cells [10] and enhances the antitumor effects of chemotherapy or irradiation in vivo and in vitro [6, 11]. To our knowledge, there has been no report concerning the effect of hyperthermia alone or of hyperthermo-chemo-radiotherapy on a human squamous cell carcinoma of the esophagus in vitro. We established a new cell line (KSE-1) from a squamous cell carcinoma derived from a human esophageal cancer [12] (Fig. 3.1). Using this cell line we attempted to clarify whether hyperthermia is an effective treatment for human squamous cell carcinoma in vitro and whether hyperthermo-chemo-radiotherapy is more effective than a single modality or two modalities.

The KSE-1 cell line was grown in Dulbecco's modified Eagle medium (DMEM) supplemented with 10% of heat-inactivated fetal calf serum and 5 µg/ml of gentamicin at 37°C in a humidified 5% CO_2/95% air atmosphere. The pH was adjusted to 7.4 by changing the gas phase concentration of CO_2 30 min prior to treatments, and was monitored throughout the course of the experiment by inserting a glass microelectrode into the medium.

Replicate plates (60 mm; Falcon) inoculated with 1×10^5 KSE-1 cells were incubated at 37°C for 48 h and the cells were used for various forms of treatment.

The number of viable cells in each dish was assayed by trypan blue dye exclusion after removal of cells with 0.25% trypsin solution. Percent cell growth was expressed by the cell number of the treated cultures

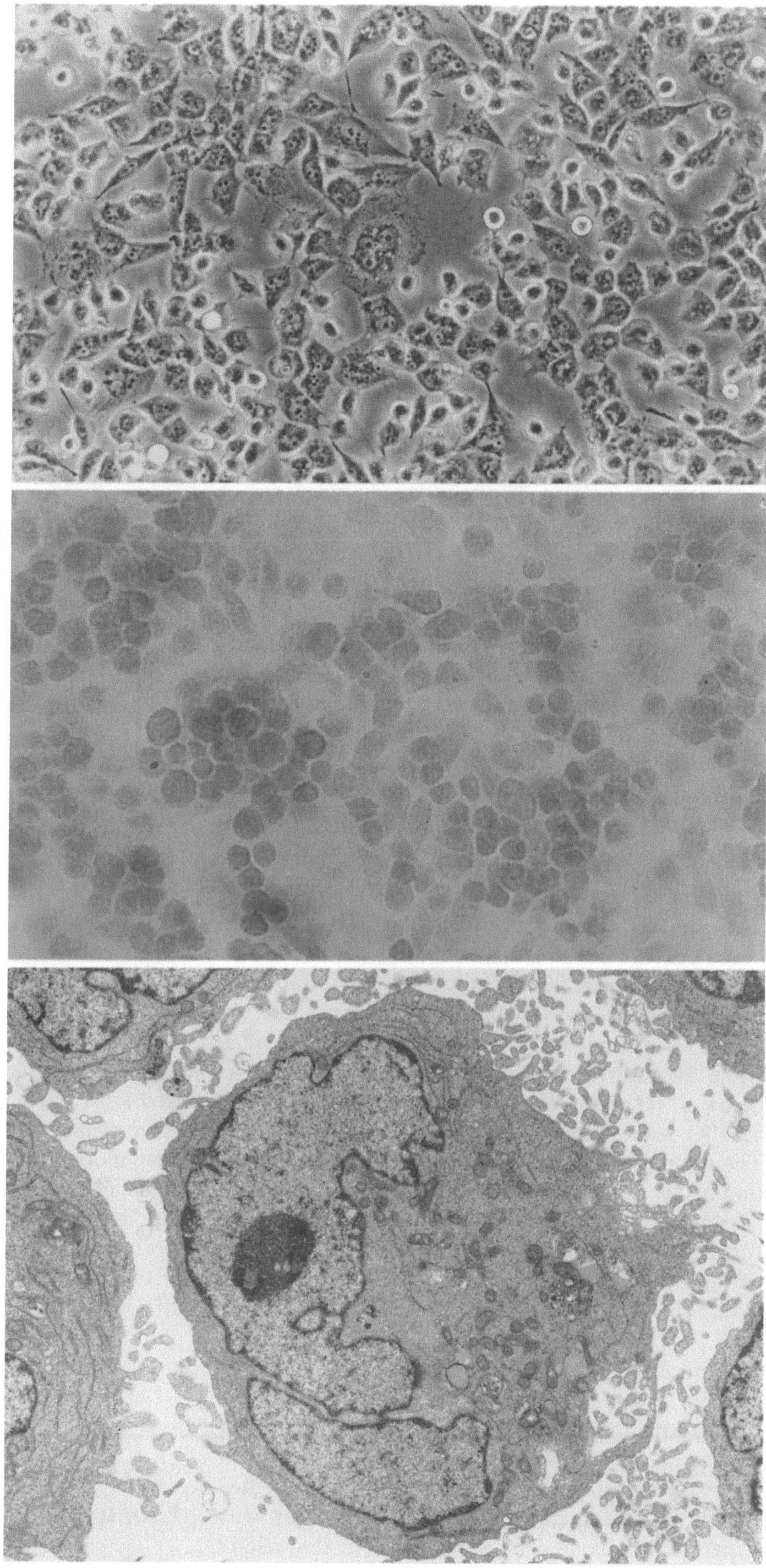

Fig. 3.1. a KSE-1 cells at the 50th passage on a double-chamber Lab-Tek slide. Spindle-shaped cells with vesicular nuclei are present. **b** The keratin staining of the cultured KSE-1 cells. The avidin-biotin-complex (ABC) method used to detect keratin was positive. ×200. **c** Electron micrograph of a trypsinized KSE-1 cell. Transmission electron microscopy of the cultured KSE-1 cells revealed that these cells possessed a number of rough endoplasmic reticuli, free and membrane-bound ribosomes, lysosomes, microvilli, and a few mitochondria. ×610000

relative to the cell numbers of untreated control cultures.

Hyperthermia was carried out at temperatures from 37 °C to 44 ° ±0.1 °C. The temperature of the medium was adjusted to the individual temperature within times from 3 to 5 min. Incubation time was from 30 to 120 min. Control cultures were incubated at 37 °C. The cells were incubated in 10% DMEM containing BLM at various concentrations from 0.002 to 200 µg/ml for 60 min at 37 °C and given X-rays from 0.5 to 2.5 Gy.

To evaluate the efficiency of the combination treatment using two or three modalities, the cells were treated as fallows:

1. Hyperthermo-chemotherapy: The cells in 10% DMEM containing BLM at a concentration of 2 µg/ml were incubated for 60 min at 42 °C
2. Hyperthermo-radiotherapy: Immediately after irradiation with 2.0 Gy, the cells were incubated at 42 °C for 60 min
3. Chemo-radiotherapy: The cells were first irradiated and thereafter incubated in 10% DMEM containing BLM at a concentration of 2 µg/ml for 60 min at 37 °C
4. Hyperthermo-chemo-radiotherapy: The cells were first irradiated in 10% DMEM and incubated for 60 min at 42 °C, immediately after adding BLM to the medium, at the final concentration of 2 µg/ml.

The response of KSE-1 cells to different temperatures and exposure to hyperthermia for various times was observed. The effect of hyperthermia was dependent on both the applied temperature and the duration of exposure. A precipitous fall in cell growth was observed at temperatures between 42° and 42.5 °C, while the growth was little affected at temperatures below 41 °C. Further elevation of temperature from 42.5 °C resulted in a slight decline in cell growth.

The responses of the KSE-1 line to a single application of hyperthermia, chemotherapy, and radiotherapy was determined. Based on these findings, in the further experiments to determine the enhanced effects of these modalities, doses which reduced the growth to approximately 80% were used in each modality, i.e., 42 °C, 60 min for hyperthermia (79.5%), 60 min for 2 µg/ml BLM solution (78.4%), and 2.0 Gy for irradiation (81.8%).

The growth rate of cells on hyperthermo-chemo-radiotherapy was the lowest among the treatments. The growth rate in the case of treatment with hyperthermo-chemo-radiotherapy was lower than that with hyperthermia alone. The growth rate in the case of hyperthermia alone was lower than that with no treatment. As shown in Table 3.2, the percent cell growth after treatment with three modalities (hyperthermo-chemo-radiotherapy) was 49%, a value much lower than that with two modalities, i.e., hyperthermo-chemotherapy, hyperthermo-radiotherapy, or chemo-radiotherapy. The differences were statistically significant ($P<0.01$).

Table 3.2. Effects of hyperthermia, chemotherapy, and irradiation on cell growth

Treatment	Percent cell growth
Single modality	
Hyperthermia	79.5 ± 9.5
Chemotherapy	78.4 ± 10.9
Radiotherapy	81.8 ± 11.8
Two modalities	
Hyperthermo-chemotherapy	70.5 ± 6.9
Hyperthermo-radiotherapy	72.1 ± 4.3
Chemo-radiotherapy	75.2 ± 3.6
Three modalities	
Hyperthermo-chemo-radiotherapy	48.5 ± 4.1

The KSE-1 cell line responded well to hyperthermia, as have other lines such as the Chinese hamster ovary [11] and the gliosarcoma cell lines [13]. The effect of hyperthermia increased with rise in temperature and incubation time.

The dose-dependent effects of hyperthermia, chemotherapy, or radiotherapy alone were also studied using the KSE-1 line. Based on these findings, the effects of combinations with subthreshold doses of each modality were examined. The effects of two modalities on KSE-1 cells were increased in comparison with those of hyperthermia alone. According to previous reports, hyperthermia enhanced the radioresponse and thus inhibited the repair of sublethal damage [6], and enhanced the cell killing by bleomycin by inhibiting the recovery from potentially lethal damage [11].

With regard to the mechanism of the effects of the three modalities, we speculate that repair of the DNA damage by radiotherapy or chemotherapy might be blocked by hyperthermia as hyperthermo-chemo-radiotherapy was more effective than a single modality or two modalities on the KSE-1 line, with statistical differences. We believe that hyperthermo-chemo-radiotherapy may prove to be an effective and reasonable adjuvant treatment for esophageal carcinoma.

3.3 Heat Delivery for Carcinoma of the Esophagus

Hyperthermia is particularly effective for the treatment of clinical carcinoma when applied concomi-

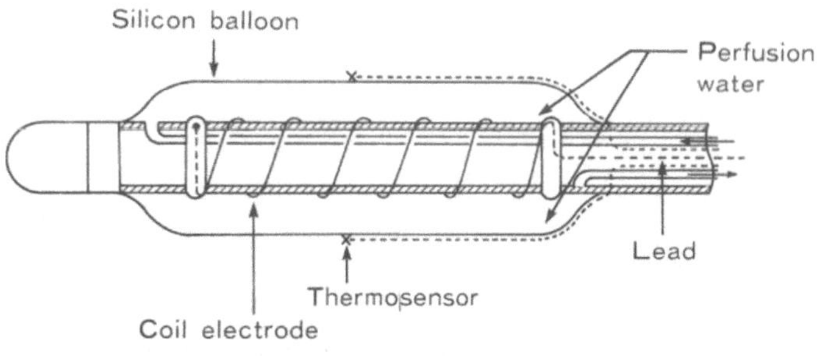

Fig. 3.2. Structure of the electrode for radiofrequency

tantly with radiation and chemotherapy [14, 15]. However, there are certain difficulties when hyperthermia is to be applied to a deeply located lesion. The approach to heating only a deep portion of the body and the measurement of the exact temperature in these deep areas have remained problematic. One of the solutions is to insert an electrode into the esophagus orally.

The difficulty in actual use is how to control the heating safely. We have to protect the treated area from being overheated or even burned by carefully monitoring the temperature. As the area of maximum heat generation is the inner surface of the esophagus, special care should be taken here.

Radiofrequency (RF) heating techniques employing capacitive electrodes have often been used in attempts to induce deep body hyperthermia [16]. RF applicators can be classified into two groups – electric and magnetic devices. In the frequency range commonly used for these methods (8–30 MHz), heating is predominantly due to conduction currents in the tissues. We devised an electrode for RF (Figs. 3.2, 3.3). When this electrode is inserted into the gastrointestinal tract, a deep portion can be properly warmed and the exact temperature monitored.

Considering the above-mentioned point, we have developed the following systems of hyperthermia for carcinoma of the esophagus. A small area electrode (an intraluminal applicator: a thin cylinder 8×80 mm) is inserted into the esophagus via the mouth and a large area electrode (an extracorporeal applicator: a rectangular sheet 100×400 mm) is attached to the body surface. Then applying the RF current between the two electrodes, the RF field concentrates near the intraluminal applicator due to the difference of area between the electrodes. In this way the esophagus can be effectively heated (Figs. 3.4, 3.5).

To apply this method to a patient, we have developed an electrode and a heating control system (Endoradiotherm 100A: Kureha Chemical Industry Co. 103 Horidome, Nihonbashi, Chuo-ku, Tokyo, Japan) (Figs. 3.6, 3.7). The main structure of the electrode consists of the fallowing three parts:

1. Transmitter for RF radiation (13.56 MHz, 250 W)
2. A balloon and a cooling system which fills the gap

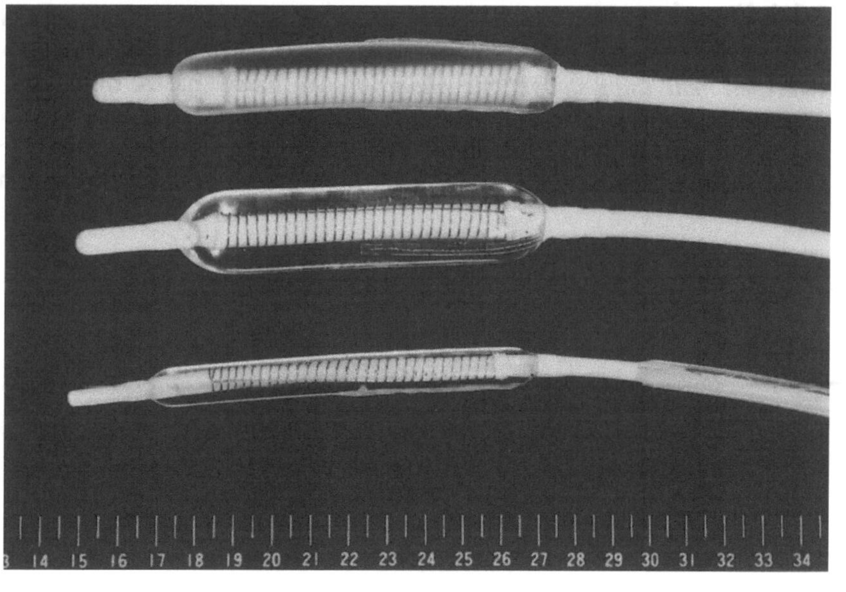

Fig. 3.3. Three types of electrode for radiofrequency

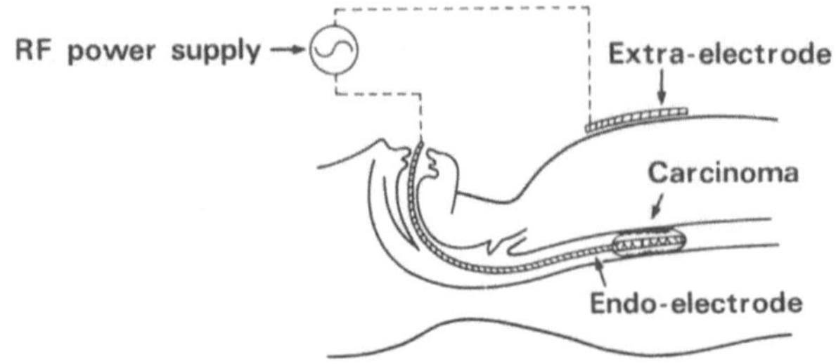

Fig. 3.4. Schema of clinical hyperthermia for esophageal carcinoma

between the malignant tissue and the transmitter with coolant: 60 ml/min of water at body temperature was circulated to prevent overheating of the transmitter

3. Thermosensor: Cooper/constantan thermocouples (IT-18, Baily Company, USA) were fixed on the outside of the balloon.

The Endoradiotherm 100A has the following features:

1. Frequency 13.56 MHz; maximum power: 250 W
2. Temperature sensing: CC thermocouple – two points
3. Heating control: ON/OFF control
4. A measurement and control interval of 1 s.

Noiseless measurement has been accomplished under the RF field. A block diagram of the Endoradiotherm 100A is shown in Fig. 3.8.

We have studied the heating characteristics around the intraluminal applicator. The first example concerns a dynamic phantom, the second, a canine gastric tube.

3.3.1 Experiments

1. Experiment using a dynamic phantom: We have prepared a simple dynamic phantom to simulate cooling by blood flow. The structure of this phantom is shown in Fig. 3.9. A mixture of Sephadex G-25 gel and 0.3 wt% NaCl solution was placed into the phantom cylinder (150∅ × 250 mm). This gel restrains water convection, and composes paths of coolant. The intraluminal applicator was fixed in the center of the cylinder and some sensors were fixed near the applicator. The extracorporeal applicator (150∅ × 100 mm) was attached on the inner surface of the cylinder. A nylon mesh was placed on the cylinder bottom. The liquid component was drawn out through the nylon mesh by persist pump (Roller Pump), and returned to the phantom cylinder top through a heat exchanger at a constant temperature. Results are shown in Fig. 3.10. Experimental results show that effective heating near the intraluminal applicator can be accomplished up to a depth of about 5–10 mm from the balloon surface, and the temperature rise near the extracorporeal applicator is negligible. Furthermore, the Endoradiotherm 100A can measure the temperature under the RF field, so we can obtain the precise curve of temperature rise and analyze the mechanism of heating and cooling in detail.

2. Experiment using the stomach of a mongrel dog: The narrowly plasticized pyloric canal of mongrel dogs was used as an experimental model for temperature assessment (Fig. 3.11). Three thermosensors were inserted into each layer of the gastric wall, and the time course of temperature during RF irradiation was measured. When measuring the temperature, the generator output was interrupted. The desired temperature range for hyperthermic treatment was readily obtained, even at 6 mm from the mucosal surface (Fig. 3.12). The exact temperature of the lesion can be obtained from the thermosensor attached to the balloon surface.

3. Heat delivery in clinical carcinoma of the esophagus: Figure 3.13a is a schematic diagram of how a carcinoma of the esophagus is warmed by the RF antenna. A thin, long electrode in the esophagus and a broad and wide counterelectrode at the body surface make possible localization of the electromagnetic field at the esophagus and provide effective heat to

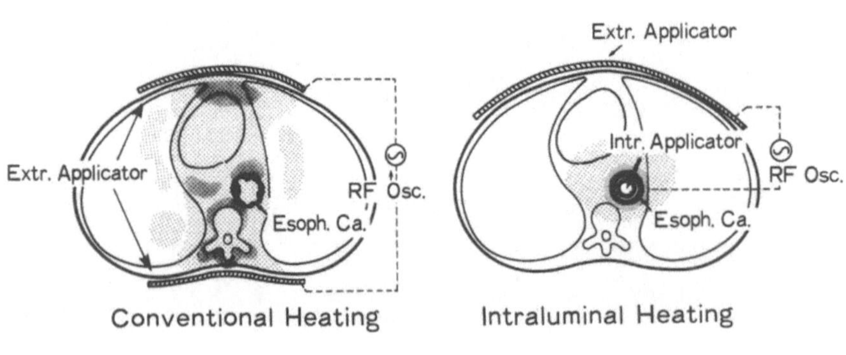

Fig. 3.5. Heating principle. *Left*: Conventional heating using two extracorporeal electrodes. *Right*: Our intraluminal heating using a combination of a large extracorporeal electrode and a small intraluminal electrode

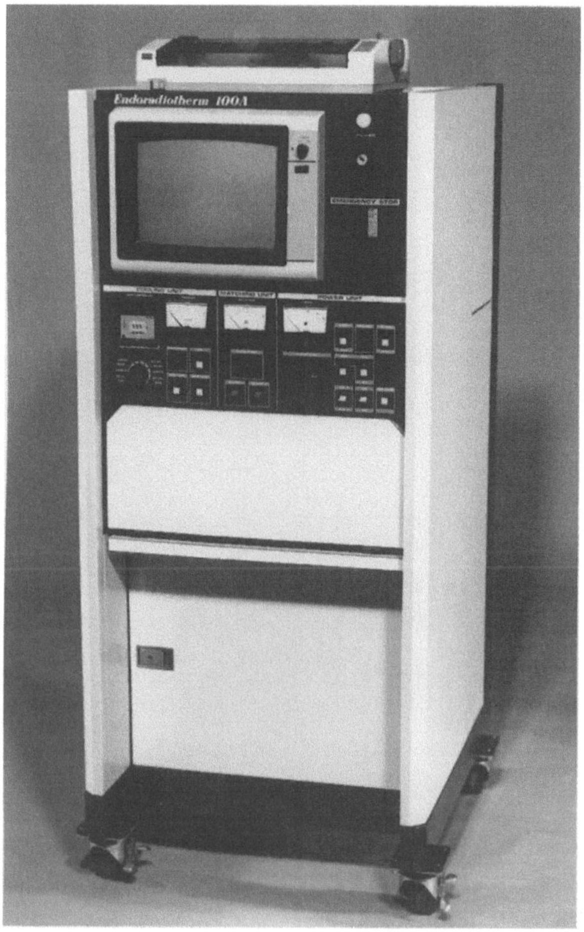

Fig. 3.6. The Endoradiotherm 100A

portions of the esophagus, which it would otherwiese not be feasible to reach. The temperature of the endotract antenna is controlled by the cooling water system within the balloon. Thermosensors attached to the balloon surface indicate the temperature of the tumor surface. By suitably rotating the counterelectrode, circumferential heating of the esophagus is feasible.

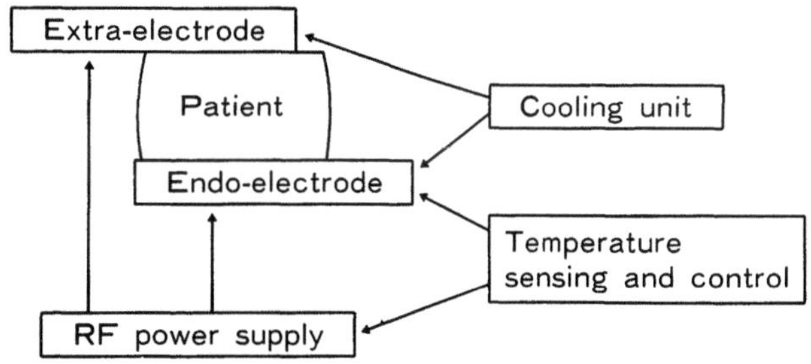

Fig. 3.7. The system construction of the heating system

We have been using these devices for 5 years in the treatment for esophageal carcinoma and have obtained good results.

Various methods of producing local and regional hyperthermia, such as regional perfusion of the extremities, water bath immersion, ultrasound, and nonionizing electromagnetic radiation, including radiofrequency and microwave radiation, have been used to investigate the efficacy of heat as a clinical modality for treating superficial cancers [17–21]. However, selective heating of deeply located malignant tissue has heretofore not been possible.

In 1978 we initiated a clinical study on esophageal carcinoma by infusing water at 55°–60°C into the esophageal balloon of a Sengstaken-Blakemore tube, usually applied a means of hemostasis for bleeding esophageal varices [15]. In six of eight patients treated with heat combined with radiation and chemotherapy the response was positive (75%). However, it was difficult to apply this system to patients with severe stenosis due to esophageal carcinoma. After several years of continued research on designs, we devised a hyperthermia electrode which can heat the deep portion of the body.

The essential conditions for clinical application of hyperthermia are: (a) safety, (b) that the entire tumor can be properly heated, (c) that the temperature of the tumor be measured accurately and controlled easily

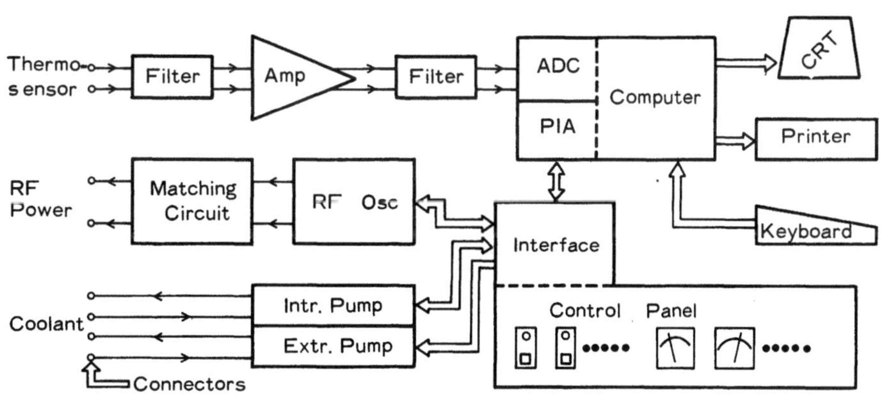

Fig. 3.8. Block diagram of the Endoradiotherm 100A

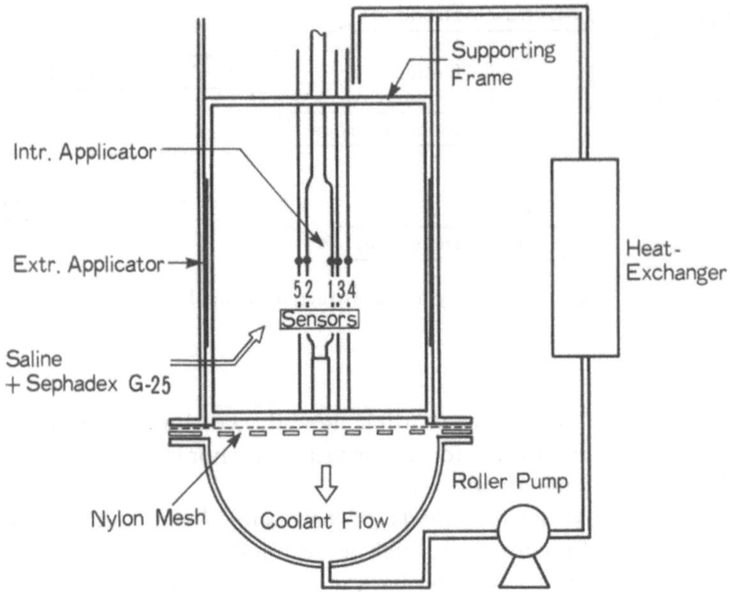

Fig. 3.9. Dynamic phantom

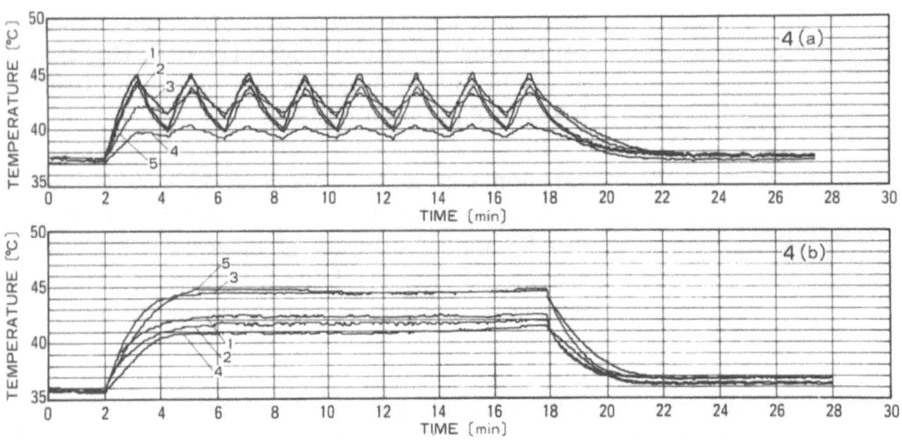

Fig. 3.10. Temperature data

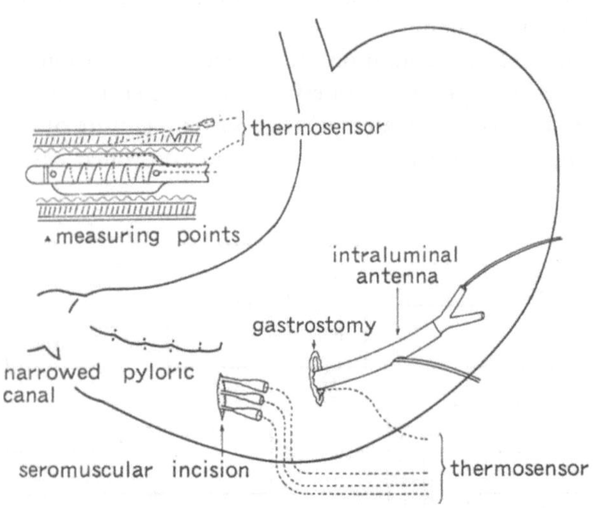

Fig. 3.11. Schema of warming. The temperature of the narrowly plasticized gastric wall of a mongrel dog was monitored at three points by the use of thermosensors

and d) that hyperthermia can be easily repeated. All of these requirements were free from danger with trials of up to a total of more than 500 fractions for patients with carcinoma of the esophagus. Employing thoracotomy, the hyperthermic zone of the outer wall of the esophagus was investigated. We found that when the mucosal, surface of the esophagus was heated to 44.5 °C, the temperature of the outer side of the tumor exceeded 42.5 °C. Thus, all the layer of the esophagus, including the malignancy, was well heated by the radiofrequency system.

The above-mentioned device, involving use of an endotract electrode, is available for use in other types of malignancy, such as colorectal carcinoma or carcinoma of the uterine cervix. Further related clinical studies are underway using this inexpensive, easy-to-use equipment to treat malignant tumors.

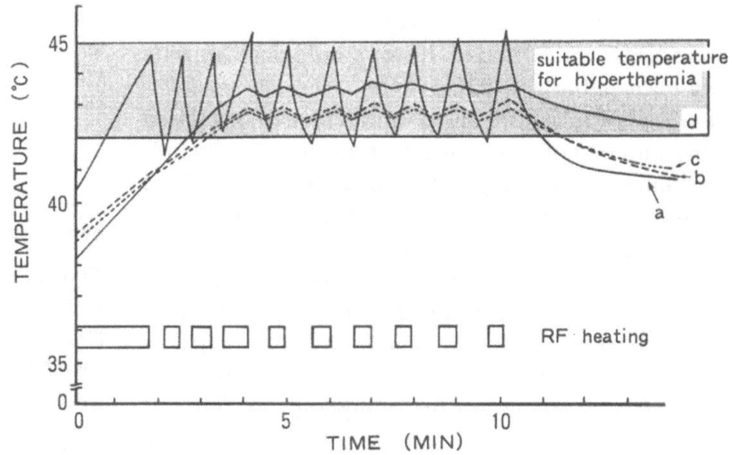

Fig. 3.12. Temperature at each depth of the gastric wall. *a*, outer surface of the balloon; *b*, 2.2 mm depth; *c*, 2.8 mm depth; *d*, subserosa (5.6 mm depth). An ideal temperature for hyperthermia was easily obtained with this electrode

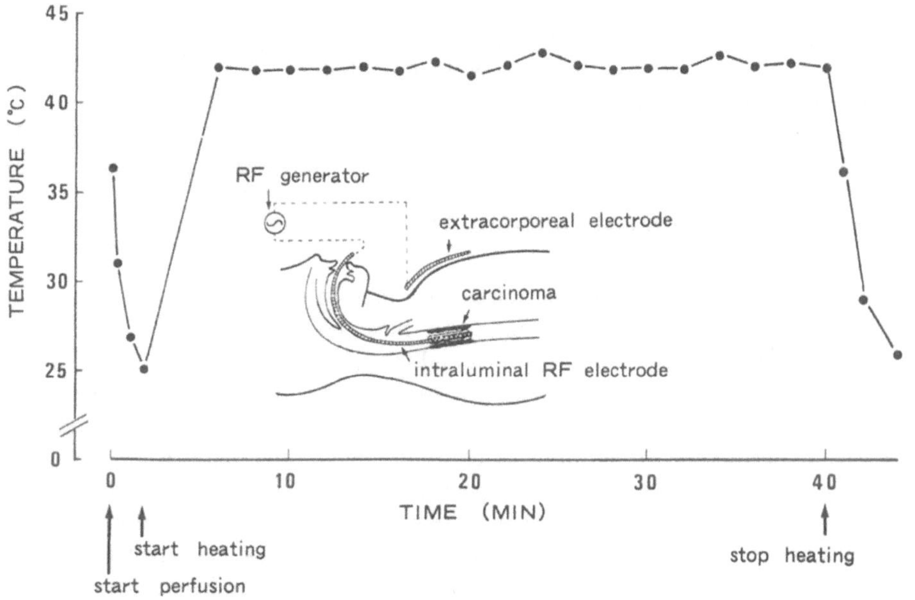

Fig. 3.13. Temperature of esophageal carcinoma heated with RF. A suitable temperature for hyperthermia treatment was obtained with a heating time of 5 min

3.4 Clinical Investigations on the Combination of Hyperthermia, Chemotherapy, and Irradiation for Carcinoma of the Esophagus

As an effective treatment for malignant tumors, hyperthermia is already being clinically applied concomitantly with irradiation and chemotherapy against superficial tumors and malignant melanomas; however, most of the reports regarding its effectiveness are indicative of the reaction of the local lesions, such as reduction of tumor volume and necrosis of tumor tissue, and the improvement in long-term results among patients treated with hyperthermia has not been reported.

In our department, hyperthermia was applied against esophageal carcinoma in 1978. Initially heating was by hot water using the Sengstaken-Blakemore balloon usually applied during bleeding from esophageal varices but later we used radiofrequency. The histopathological changes in eight resected specimens of carcinoma of the esophagus subjected to concomitant application of hyperthermia, irradiation, and chemotherapy before surgery have been reported [15]. In 1979, esophageal heating by intraluminal microwave was applied to many patients with esophageal carcinoma, and detailed histopathological reports have been published [22].

Microwave applicators based on microstrip or related techniques can offer a number of advantages, including small size, low weight, and the ability to conform to tissue surfaces; however, penetration into tissues is relatively poor. On the other hand, in 1983, a sophisticated electrode for radiofrequency, to be inserted into the esophagus, was developed which made the esophageal heating easier and reliable [23]. Generally, as the capacity of the microwave to heat the deeply located tissues is less powerful compared to that of radiofrequency, the latter is more suitable in heating carcinoma of the esophagus, the rectum, etc., while microwave is applied in heating rather small carcinomas.

In this paper, the histophathological efficacy of hyperthermia, the long-term results, and the sensitivity of the esophageal cancer cells to heating will be presented.

Table 3.3. Relationship between treatment methods and pathological manifestations

Lesion	Treatment			Control
	IMH	IMH plus RT[a]	RT	
Superficial necrosis	10/10	8/8	8/10	5/10
Necrosis of paracancer epithelium	8/10	7/8	7/10	0
Necrosis at edge of cancer nest	8/10	8/8	5/10	1/10
Round cell reaction				
Slight	2/10	3/11	8/10	2/10
Moderate	5/10	4/11	2/10	0
Considerable or marked	3/10	4/11	0	0
Interstitial widening	3/10	8/11	8/10	2/10
Capillary congestion	10/10	8/8	8/10	4/10
Capillary stasis	10/10	8/8	6/10	0
Capillary hemorrhage	5/10	6/8	5/10	0
Necrosis of capillary wall	6/10	6/8	4/10	0

IMH, intraluminal microwave hyperthermia; RT, radiation therapy
[a] Three patients "void of cancer" were not included

3.4.1 Histophathological Evaluation

There are a few reports of histopathological studies in patients with esophageal carcinoma who have received hyperthermia. Qui et al. [22] reviewed the specimens from 21 patients who underwent esophagectomy and who had been treated with intraluminal microwave hyperthermia either alone or combined with radiotherapy. The controls were ten surgical specimens from patients who had been treated with 3000–4000 rad only and another ten who had no therapy before resection.

From the preliminary analysis, one can conclude that the differences were substantial in the therapeutic reactions between hyperthermia groups and control groups, and between hyperthermia plus radiation and radiation groups. They showed that the histopathological changes in the hyperthermia and the control groups were different (Table 3.3). However, these differences were not dramatic in all the treatment groups. No specific reaction has been identified as being a hyperthermia-induced one. Sugaar and Leveen [24] regarded interstitial vascular fibrinoid necrosis and the numerous small round cell infiltrations as specific post-hyperthermic lesions.

As we have already reported [25], histopathological evaluation of hyperthermo-chemo-radiotherapy (HCR) for carcinoma of the esophagus was carried out. One hundred and seventy-eight Japanese pa-

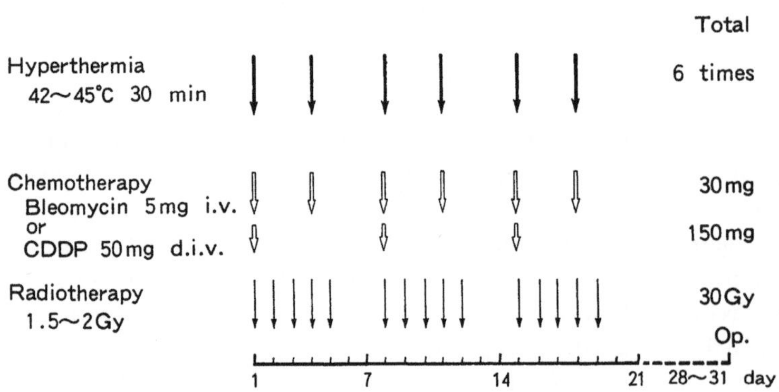

Fig. 3.14. Regimen of HCR

Table 3.4. Clinical data in 178 Japanese patients with esophageal carcinoma

	Group I	Group II	Total
Patients	116 (100)[a]	62 (100)	178 (100)
Sex (n, %)			
Male	100 (86.2)	55 (88.7)	155 (87.1)
Female	16 (13.8)	7 (11.3)	23 (12.9)
Age (yr)			
Range	46 – 80	38 – 81	38 – 81
Mean	56.2 ± 7.8	62.0 ± 8.4	58.2 ± 8.4
Site of carcinoma			
Upper esophagus	12 (10.3)	12 (19.4)	24 (13.5)
Mid-esophagus	78 (67.2)	37 (59.7)	115 (64.6)
Lower esophagus	26 (22.4)	13 (21.0)	39 (21.9)

[a] ( ), percent

tients with esophageal carcinoma underwent esophageal resection and reconstruction.

The regimen of HCR used by us is shown in Fig. 3.14. Irradiation with ^{60}Co or X-ray was given in a dose of 1.5 – 2.0 Gy per day, five times a week. Hyperthermia was initiated at 42 °– 45 °C for 30 min, and given twice a week. This hyperthermia was initiated within an hour after termination of irradiation. Chemotherapy using bleomycin 5 mg i.v. was performed simultaneously with hyperthermia. Such HCR therapy was continued for 3 weeks with a total of 30 Gy irradiation, 30 mg bleomycin, and six exposures to hyperthermia; all patients tolerated this preoperative treatment well. About two weeks after termination of HCR, esophageal resection and reconstruction were carried out.

One hundred and sixteen patients (group I) were treated with chemotherapy and irradiation between 25 and 35 Gy preoperatively. Sixty-two other patients (group II) underwent surgery after preoperative HCR (Table 3.4).

The histological effectiveness of the preoperative therapy was studied in the resected tissues. In patients in whom viable neoplastic cells were completely destroyed the treatment was defined as "markedly effective," while in patients in whom most of cancer cells were extensively damaged, despite the presence of a few viable cells, it was defined as "moderately effective". In all other treatments was categorized as "ineffective." These criteria were defined and published by the Japanese Society of Esophageal Diseases [26]. There were 14 (12.1%) patients in group I and 14 (22.6%) in group II in whom no viable cancer cells were found (markedly effective treatment), while in 43 (37.1%) patients in group I and 27 (43.5%) in group II treatment was classed as moderately effective (Table 3.5).

Table 3.5. Histological effectiveness of preoperative combined therapy

Histological effectiveness	Group I (116 cases)	Group II (62 cases)	Total
Ineffective	59 (50.9)	21 (33.9)	80 (44.9)
Moderately effective	43 (37.1)	27 (43.5)	70 (39.3)
Markedly effective	14 (12.1)	14 (22.6)	28 (15.7)
Total	116 (100)	62 (100)	178 (100)

Table 3.6. Survival rates in patients receiving HCR or CR therapy preoperatively

Group	No. of patients	Survival rate (%) 1 yr	2 yrs	3 yrs	4 yrs	5 yrs
HCR	62	65.8	50.4	43.2	43.2	43.2
CR	121	44.9	26.9	20.4	16.6	14.7

Although the number of patients treated with preoperative HCR has been only 62, this approach nevertheless shows great promise in patients with esophageal cancer.

3.4.2 Long-term Results

We have clinically applied HCR since 1978. Here we describe our long-term results in patients with esophageal carcinoma who received hyperthermia: to our knowledge, there have been no previous reports of long-term results in patients who have received hyperthermia.

Sixty-two patients had received preoperative HCR and an other 121 had been treated with irradiation and chemotherapy preoperatively (CR therapy).

In the majority of patients, the operation was carried out in one stage; subtotal esophagectomy and lymph node dissection were performed through a right thoracotomy and esophageal reconstruction was carried out with a gastric tube via the antesternal route [27].

The regimen of preoperative HCR in patients with resectable carcinoma was as described in the previous section.

Table 3.6 shows the survival rates of patients who received preoperative HCR or preoperative CR (the

Table 3.7. Survival rates of patients with stage I or II resectable carcinoma

Group	No. of patients	Survival rate (%)				
		1 yr	2 yrs	3 yrs	4 yrs	5 yrs
HCR	35	70.6	64.8	55.5	–	–
CR	53	60.1	38.2	30.2	26.1	24.0

Table 3.8. Survival rates of patients with stage III or IV resectable carcinoma

Group	No. of patients	Survival rate (%)				
		1 yr	2 yrs	3 yrs	4 yrs	5 yrs
HCR	27	62.5	37.9	37.9	37.9	37.9
CR	68	31.5	16.5	10.5	7.5	6.0

Table 3.9. Survival rates of patients with unresectable carcinoma

Group	No. of patients	Survival rate (%)			
		0.5 yrs	1 yr	1.5 yrs	2 yrs
HCR	31	62.6	33.2	20.7	15.5
CR	83	54.2	10.8	1.2	1.2

Table 3.10. Survival rates of patients with stage I or II unresectable carcinoma

Group	No. of patients	Survival rate (%)			
		0.5 yrs	1 yr	1.5 yrs	2 yrs
HCR	14	87.5	61.4	40.9	27.3
CR	29	69.0	20.7	3.4	3.4

Table 3.11. Survival rates of patients with stage III or IV unresectable carcinoma

Group	No. of patients	Survival rate (%)			
		0.5 yrs	1 yr	1.5 yrs	2 yrs
HCR	17	40.7	16.3	8.1	8.1
CR	54	46.3	5.6	0	0

control group). Two-year survival rates in the HCR group and the control group were 50.4% and 26.9%, respectively. Survival rates in patients who received HCR were significantly better than those in patients who received CR preoperatively ($P<0.05$).

Table 3.7 shows the survival rates in patients with TNM stages I and II who were treated surgically, while Table 3.8 shows those in patients with TNM stages III and IV. In the latter group survival rates were statistically significantly better in patients given preoperative HCR ($P<0.05$).

There were an other 114 patients none of whom had undergone resection of the esophageal carcinoma. These patients were divided into two groups according to treatment status. Of these patients, 31 received HCR and 83 CR. Far advanced tumorous processes and associated severe diseases were the main reasons why resection could not be performed.

There were no significant differences between the groups with regard to prognostic factors such as age, sex, site of carcinoma, and TNM stage.

For patients with unresectable carcinoma of the esophagus, the same regimen of HCR was prescribed and was continued as many times as possible. Average doses of each modality were as follows: 12.3 applications of hyperthermia, 46.9 Gy irradiation (X-rays) and 30.7 mg bleomycin. The average doses of irradiation and chemotherapy for patients with unresectable carcinoma who were treated with irradiation and chemotherapy without hyperthermia were 48.5 Gy and 38.2 mg bleomycin, respectively. There was no statistical difference between the groups with regard to doses of irradiation and chemotherapy.

Table 3.9 shows survival rates in the patients with unresectable carcinoma of the esophagus. Survival rates at 12 months in patients who received HCR and CR were 33.2% and 10.8%, respectively, while those at 24 months were 15.5% and 1.2% respectively. There is a statistical difference in favor of HCR as compared with CR ($P<0.05$). Overall, the median survival was 9.5 months for patients receiving HCR and 6.1 months for patients receiving CR.

The survival rates according to the TNM stage in patients with unresectable carcinoma are shown in Tables 3.10 and 3.11. Although there were no statistical differences in survival rates in those with stages III and IV, among the patients classified having as stage I and II disease, the survival rates of patients who received HCR were significantly better than those of patients who received CR ($P<0.05$). The mean survival time of stage I and II patients given HCR was 14.4 months, whereas that of patients given CR without hyperthermia was only 8.6 months.

As we have already reported [28], when cancer cells of the esophagus were strongly damaged preoperatively, the 5-year survival rate of patients who received surgery was 45.1%. These findings suggest that it is very important to increase the direct effect of irradiation on cancer cells before surgery.

Our data suggest that proper hyperthermia combined with radiation and chemotherapy shows great promise in the treatment of patients with esophageal carcinoma. As local hyperthermia has no severe side-effects, this treatment is thought to be one of the most interesting modalities to be considered in patients with malignant lesions such as carcinoma of the esophagus. We also consider that our intracavital radiofrequency applicator is one solution to problems of clinical application of hyperthermia for carcinoma of the esophagus.

3.4.3 Multi-institutional Report

We have tentatively undertaken multi-institutional study involving 13 surgical teams who have been treating esophageal carcinoma, and a cooperative study was undertaken to assess the usefulness and efficacy of hyperthermia in carcinoma of the esophagus.

As shown in Figs. 3.3 and 3.6, the Endoradiotherm 100A was used. Side-effects such as a local heat sensation and pyrexia occurred in about 10% of patients; however, these effects were transient and mild, and no patients could not tolerate hyperthermia treatment.

Seventy-nine Japanese patients with primary esophageal carcinoma underwent hyperthermia treatment between August 1984 and August 1985 in 13 institutions[1] in Japan. These patients were divided into two groups, based on the resectability of the lesion. Group A comprised 38 patients who underwent subtotal esophagectomy after preoperative hyperthermia plus chemotherapy and/or radiotherapy (HCR therapy). Group B comprised 41 patients not treated surgically who received hyperthermia alone or with irradiation and/or chemotherapy. The related data are shown in Table 3.12.

[1] Participants in this study: K. Sugimachi, The 2nd Department of Surgery, Faculty of Medicine, Kyushu University, K. Isono; The 2nd Department of Surgery, School of Medicine, Chiba University; M. Kasai, The 2nd Department of Surgery, School of Medicine, Tohoku University; T. Uchino, The 1st Department of Surgery, School of Medicine, Hokkaido University; O. Abe, Department of Surgery, School of Medicine, Keio University; M. Endo, Department of Surgery, Gastointestinal Disease Center, Tokyo Women's Medical College; K. Nabeya, The 2nd Department of Surgery School of Medicine, Kyorin University; T. Mitomi, The 2nd Department of Surgery, School of Medicine, Tokai University; T. Muto, The 1st Department of Surgery, School of Medicine, Niigata University; T. Hattori, Department of Surgery, Research Institute for Nuclear Medicine and Biology, Hiroshima University; S. Koga, The 1st Department of Surgery, School of Medicine, Tottori University; T. Nakamura, The 2nd Department of Surgery, Shimane Medical College; M. Kobayashi, The 1st Department of Surgery, Oita Medical College

Table 3.12. Clinical data in 79 Japanese patients with primary esophageal carcinoma who underwent hyperthermia treatment

	Group A: surgical cases (38 patients)	Group B: unresectable cases (41 patients)
Age (years)		
Range	42–78	49–83
Mean	63.2	67.3
Sex		
Male	32	38
Female	6	3
Size of tumor (cm)		
Mean	6.4	6.4
Range	1.5–13.0	1.1–13.0

Table 3.13. Details of combined therapy

Therapy	Group A: surgical cases (38 patients)	Group B: unresectable cases (41 patients)
HCR	25	20
HR	4	12
HC	8	9
H	1	

Abbreviations for all tables: HCR, hyperthermochemoradiotherapy; HR, hyperthermo-radiotherapy; HC, hyperthermo-chemotherapy; H, hyperthermia

In the group A patients with resectable carcinoma, preoperative HCR was given for 3 weeks at 3 or 4 day intervals for a total of six times. The range of temperature was controlled from 42° to 45 °C for 30 min. Hyperthermia was begun within 1 h after the cessation of radiation therapy, each of which about 2.0 Gy reached 30 Gy. Chemotherapy was given concomitantly with the hyperthermia. Bleomycin and cis-platinum were the drugs mainly prescribed, and they were selected by the attending physicians in each institute. In group B patients is whom esophagectomy was not indicated, HCR was given. The doses given exceeded those in group A, reaching 46.6 Gy radiation and 12.5 applications of hyperthermia on average. The combined therapy was as shown in Table 3.13.

Clinical efficacy based on the tumor regression was determined by radiographs and endoscopic findings were assessed according to the guidelines for clinical and pathological studies on solid tumors [29]. In the instances of disappearance of all recognized disease, the treatment was considered to have achieved a complete response (CR). When a 50% or more decrease (two dimensions) or a 30% or more decrease (single dimension) in total tumor size was achieved, the treatment effect was adjudged to be a partial response (PR). In cases of a less than 50% decrease (two dimensions) in the size of the tumor (or a less than 30% decrease on the single dimension), the treatment effect was considered to be no change (NC). With a 25% or more increase in the size of the lesion, or the appearance of new lesions, the verdict was progressive disease (PD).

Histological studies of the resected specimens were also based on defined criteria [26] and the therapy was classified as "markedly effective," "moderately effective," or "ineffective."

In addition to the objective response, the subjective symptoms were compared pre- and posttreatment. Complications such as caumesthesia, nausea, vomiting, dysorexia, and pyrexia were also evaluated, depending on the subjective complaints.

Statistical analyses were performed using Student's *t*-test.

The rates of tumor regression as evaluated by fluoroscopy and endoscopy are shown in Tables 3.14 and 3.15, respectively. In general, endoscopic examination showed a slightly better response than was seen with fluoroscopy. In the HCR group, which constituted about 70% of all cases, both examinations showed a CR or PR of about 80%. HC or H only appeared less effective than HR, which seemed about as effective as HCR. Group B showed a slightly better response than did group A. This may be due to the more frequent application of HCR in the former. Overall, combination therapy involving hyperthermia resulted in tumor regression in 60%–70% in group A and 70%–80% in group B.

In 25 patients in group A treated with HCR, treatment was "markedly effective" in 2 (8%), "moderately effective" in 15 (60%), and "ineffective" in 8 (32%), in contrast to figures of 2 of 4 (50%), 1 of 4 (25%), and 1 of 4 (25%) respectively, in patients treated with HR alone (Table 3.16). Considering all series, "markedly effective" treatment was seen in 15.8% (6/38), "moderately effective" treatment in 47.4% (18/38), and "ineffective" treatment in 36.8% (14/38). The total response rate, assumed to cover the categories "markedly effective" and "moderately effective", was thus 63.2% (24/38).

Table 3.14. Response rates evaluated by fluoroscopy

Modality	Response			
	CR	PR	NC	PD
Group A[a] (35 cases)				
HCR (25 cases)	1 (4.0)	19 (76.0)	5 (20.0)	0
	20 (80.0)			
HR (4 cases)	3	0	1	0
HC (5 cases)	0	0	5	0
H (1 cases)	0	0	1	0
Total	4 (11.4)	19 (54.3)	12 (34.3)	0
	23 (65.7)			
Group B[b] (37 cases)				
HCR (18 cases)	4 (22.2)	10 (55.5)	4 (22.2)	0
	14 (77.8)			
HR (11 cases)	6	3	2	0
HC (8 cases)	0	4	4	0
Total	10 (27.0)	17 (45.9)	10 (27.0)	0
	27 (72.9)			

Numbers in parentheses are percentages
CR, complete response; PR, partial response; NC, no change; PD, progressive disease
[a] Evaluation was not feasible in three cases
[b] Evaluation was not feasible in four cases

Table 3.15. Response rates evaluated by endoscopy

Modality	Response			
	CR	PR	NC	PD
Group A[a] (32 cases)				
HCR (24 cases)	5 (20.8)	14 (58.3)	5 (20.8)	0
	19 (79.2)			
HR (3 cases)	2	1	0	0
HC (4 cases)	0	1	3	0
H (1 case)	0	0	1	0
Total	7 (21.9)	16 (50.0)	9 (28.1)	0
	23 (71.9)			
Group B[b] (39 cases)				
HCR (18 cases)	5 (27.7)	11 (61.1)	2 (11.1)	0
	16 (88.9)			
HR (12 cases)	6	6	0	0
HC (9 cases)	0	6	3	0
Total	11 (28.2)	23 (59.0)	5 (12.8)	0
	34 (87.2)			

Numbers in parentheses are percentages
CR, complete response; PR, partial response; NC, no change; PD, progressive disease
[a] Evaluation was not feasible in six cases
[b] Evaluation was not feasible in two cases

Table 3.16. Histopathological evaluation of resected specimens (group A: 38 cases)

Modality	Markedly effective	Moderately effective	Ineffective
HCR (25)	2	15	8
HR (4)	2	1	1
HC (8)	2	2	4
H (1)	0	0	1
Total	6 (15.8%)	18 (47.4%)	14 (36.8%)

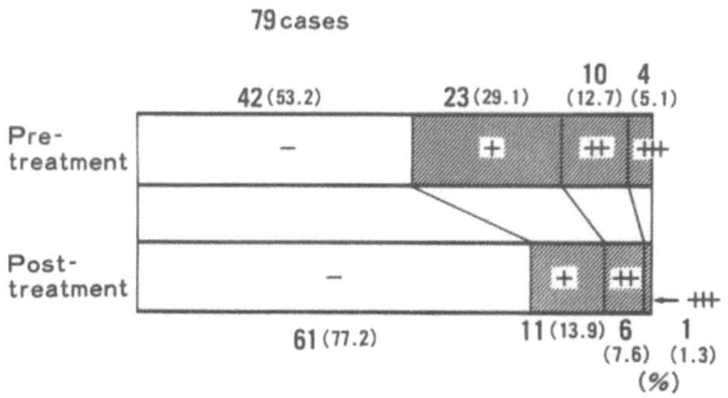

Fig. 3.15. Amelioration of dysphagia. After HCR, rates of dysphagia were markedly reduced. Dysphagia: –, none; +, mild: ++, moderate; +++, severe

The amelioration of subjective symptoms of dysphagia was marked, as shown in Fig. 3.15. The frequency of dysphagia was significantly reduced from 46.8% before treatment to 22.8% after treatment. The complications caused by Endoradiotherm 100A were minimal and transitory, and included caumesthesia (18.9%) and elevated body temperature (12.7%) (Table 3.17).

The essential conditions for clinical application – (a) safety; (b) that the entire tumor can be properly heated; (c) that the temperature of the tumor can be measured accurately and controlled easily; and (d) that hyperthermia can be easily repeated – have been ascertained to exist in the present study using our hyperthermia system in various institutions with trials a total of 459 fractions in 79 patients.

The response rates evaluated by fluoroscopy and endoscopy in both resectable and unresectable cases were 69% (50/72) and 80% (57/71), respectively. As stated above, in patients in whom carcinomas of the esophagus were excised, we confirmed histopathologically that all the viable cancer cells were completely destroyed (markedly effective treatment) in 6 of 38 cases (15.8%). Iizuka et al. [30] reported in their cooperative study that preoperative chemo-radiotherapy given to 79 patients resulted in complete destruction of cancer cells in seven (8.9%). With HCR the rate of markedly effective treatment was higher than with CR.

Table 3.17. Mild, transient complications occurring with HCR therapy using Endoradiotherm 100A

Complications	No. of patients (total: 19)
Caumesthesia	15 (18.9%)
Nausea, vomiting	5 (6.3%)
Dysorexia	2 (2.5%)
Fever	10 (12.7%)

The immediate improvement of objective findings evaluated by fluoroscopy and endoscopy, and the reduction or elimination of the lesion, are so marked that HCR using an Endoradiotherm 100 A system shows promise as a modality for treating esophageal carcinoma.

3.4.4 Hyperthermia Sensitivity Test

The biological effects of hyperthermia have been investigated using cultured cells and normal and tumoral animal tissues. Hyperthermia affect respiration and DNA, RNA, and protein synthesis in Novikoff hepatoma cells to a greater extent than is seen in the regenerating liver cells [31, 32]. There are reports indicating that transformed cells are more sensitive to treatment with 42.5 °–43 °C hyperthermia than are their normal counterparts, in vitro [33–35]. To investigate further the difference in the heat sensitivity between human tumor and normal cells, we examined changes in cell viability following exposure to a 43 °C temperature of 23 human neoplastic and adjacent normal tissues [36]. The in vitro succinate dehydrogenase inhibition (SDI) test was used [37, 38]. As the clinical effect of hyperthermia varies with the patient [39, 40], it is advisable to determine the heat sensitivity of each tumor tissue in order to improve the effectiveness of hyperthermia.

Solid tumor and adjacent normal mucosal tissues from 23 Japanese patients (15 gastric cancers and 8 colorectal cancers) were obtained at the time of gastrectomy or colectomy.

Tumor and normal tissues were cut with scissors and passed through a no. 32 stainless steel mesh into McCoy's 5A solution containing antibiotics, then washed three times with this solution. The fragments were suspended in minimal essential medium (MEM) (Nissui Seiyaku Co., Japan) with *L*-glutamine (292 mg/ml), 10% fetal calf serum (GIBCO Laboratories, USA), penicillin (100 U/ml), streptomycin (100 µg/ml), and gentamicin (40 µg/ml), plated in 35 mm plastic dishes and incubated at 37 °C (control) or 43 °C (heat treatment) in a humidified 5% CO_2 atmosphere for 20 h. Five gastric cancers and adjacent normal tissue were used to determine changes in the SD activity, following exposure to heat for 5, 10, 15, or 20 h. 3 (4,5-dimethyl-2-thiazolyl)-2,5-diphenyl-2H tetrazolium bromide (MTT) [41, 42] was used as the hydrogen acceptor for the SD activity. The formazan derived from MTT was extracted with acetone containing 0.5% trichloroacetic acid and the absorbance of formazan was measured at 565 nm. The SD

Table 3.18. Changes in SD activity of five gastric cancers and adjacent normal tissue following exposure to heat treatment for various times

Time	Tumor	Normal tissue
5[a]	93.4 ± 4.3[b]	96.8 ± 2.8[b]
10	79.1 ± 9.1	89.8 ± 5.6
15	60.6 ± 14.7	76.2 ± 9.9
20	29.8 ± 8.0	50.2 ± 11.4

[a] Incubation time (h) at 43 °C
[b] Mean ± SD

Table 3.19. Percentages of SD activity following exposure to heat treatment for 20 h in 23 tumors and adjacent normal tissue

Case	SD activity	
	Tumor	Normal tissue
Stomach		
1	7.2[a]	42.5[a]
2	15.0	41.3
3	17.0	52.1
4	18.6	42.0
5	19.3	46.4
6	25.3	39.7
7	27.4	43.8
8	31.5	59.3
9	32.1	51.8
10	34.6	48.2
11	37.2	76.2
12	40.4	61.9
13	48.7	62.3
14	53.8	58.6
15	61.6	72.6
Mean	31.3 ± 14.8[b]	53.2 ± 11.1[b]
Colon and rectum		
1	18.7	48.3
2	22.3	48.7
3	23.1	37.5
4	25.4	39.8
5	34.8	51.2
6	43.3	63.1
7	47.5	60.5
8	53.0	57.6
Mean	33.5 ± 12.2	50.8 ± 8.7

[a] Percentage of SD activity
[b] Mean ± SD

activity was presented as the optical density (OD) per milligram protein, determined using the Bio-Rad protein assay. The tumor fragments with an OD of 0.5 were plated in separate dishes. Decrease in cell viability, as induced by heat treatment, was estimated by the percentage of SD activity of the 43 °C-treated cells, compared to that of control cells, at each time.

The SD activity decreased to a greater extent in the gastric cancers than in the adjacent normal tissue, in a time-dependent fashion, as shown in Table 3.18. Significant differences were noted between the SD activities of the tumor and adjacent normal tissue: $P < 0.05$ for 15 h, $P < 0.05$ for 20 h.

The decrease in SD activity of 23 tumors was compared with that of the adjacent normal tissue, fallowing exposure to heat treatment for 20 h. As shown in Table 3.19, the SD activity decreased to a greater extent in the tumors than in the adjacent normal tissue, in each case. The means ± standard deviations of SD activity were 31.3% ± 14.8% for the gastric cancers and 53.2% ± 11.1% for the adjacent gastric normal tissue, and 33.5% ± 12.2% for the colorectal cancers and 50.8% ± 8.7% for the adjacent colorectal normal tissue. Significant differences were noted between the SD activities of the tumor and the adjacent normal tissue: $P < 0.01$ for stomach, $P < 0.05$ for colon and rectum.

To evaluate the effectiveness of hyperthermia in a clinical setting, we compared the heat sensitivity of human tumor tissue with that of adjacent normal tissue, using the SDI test. This test has been used to predict the in vitro chemosensitivity of human tumor tissues, based on correlation of the SD activity, using tetrazolium salt as the hydrogen acceptor, with the cell viability [37, 38]. We reported that the change in viability of cells exposed to antitumor drugs in the SDI test correlated with that using the in vitro ATP assay [43] and the in vivo subrenal capsule assay [44].

The heat sensitivity of human tissues was assayed in whole cells (living plus dead cells), and we determined the heat sensitivity of human tissues following long-term (20 h) incubation at 43 °C. In this condition, we found that the heat sensitivity of the tumor tissue was higher than that of adjacent normal tissue, in each case. These results correlate with the evidence that tumor cells, transformed by carcinogens [33, 34] or SV-40 [35], are more sensitive to heat treatment than are the normal counterparts. The molecular mechanism involved in the heat-induced cell killing seems to be the structural alteration of cellular DNA and DNA strand breakage (45, 46]. As the DNA synthesis and replication are more active in tumor than in normal tissues [47, 48], cellular DNA of the tumor tissues is more likely to be damaged by heat treatment, compared to events in normal tissues.

The clinical effect of hyperthermia varies between patients [39, 40]; hence the level of heat sensitivity of tumor tissue is a good index for predicting the effect of hyperthermia. As the malignant human tumor tissues were consistently more sensitive to heat than the adjacent noninvolved tissue, hyperthermia has tumor tissue selectivity as cancer therapy.

3.5 Prospects of Hyperthermia

Hyperthermia has a long tradition as a modality for treating patients with various diseases. The objective of hyperthermia for cancer patients is to destroy the malignant tissues while minimizing damage to the normal tissues.

Biological studies done in many institutes favor the clinical application of hyperthermia in combined modalities. To comprehend the action and mechanisms of hyperthermia and to develop optimal therapy modalities, biological phenomena as well as molecular, metabolic, and physiological events have to be considered. Several thousand patients have been treated with hyperthermia, in various regimens, since the 1970s. As the antitumor effect of hyperthermia alone will not suffice, combination with radiation and chemotherapy is generally prescribed.

With regard to regression of superficial tumors, the combination of radiotherapy and hyperthermia is superior to radiation alone. On the other hand, heating of deep-seated tumors, such as esophageal, liver, lung, and pancreatic cancers remains a complex technical problem. It is a challenge for physicists and engineers to design heating systems which allow safe application of heat to deep body areas, at temperatures of 42°–43°C. The required temperatures should be maintained for at least 30 min and include the complete tumor volume regardless of its shape.

Complete heating and exact measurement of the temperature, particularly in the case of carcinoma of the esophagus, meet with considerable difficulties and related research is ongoing. While, as stated above, it is technically difficult to selectively heat a deeply located tumor, to measure the temperature of the deep part noninvasively is even more difficult. Although our instrument, the Endoradiotherm 100A , will not heat a solid organ such as the liver or kidney, body cavities such as the esophagus and the rectum can be heated by insertion of the instrument.

Concerning heat resistance and heat sensitivity, basic research on heat shock protein has progressed remarkably; however, the mechanism has not been clarified. Some but not all tumors are most sensitive to hyperthermia. For a reliable comparison of the results of hyperthermia, there has to be a consensus of opinion on the thermal dose. However, at present there are no definitions of a unit of thermal dose. In the clinical application of hyperthermia, the thermal dose is vital. Are there any differences between heating at 44 °C for 30 min and heating at 43 °C for 60 min? How can the dose of heating be expressed? Moreover, it is difficult to heat different lesions using the same temperature.

In conclusion, methods of deep heating have to be improved, the possibility of noninvasive thermometry has to be considered, heat sensitivity needs to be defined, and a practical concept of thermal dose has to be worked out.

The recent wide clinical use of hyperthermia will no doubt lead to well-defined clinical trials which will provide important biological answers to hyperthermia-related problems. The design of large multicenter randomized clinical trials is to be encouraged in order to evaluate the effects of hyperthermia as primary treatment of a malignancy, with supplementary studies on metastatic and/or recurrent malignancy.

References

1. Kai H, Matsufuji H, Sugimachi K, Okudaira Y, Inokuchi K (1986) Combined effects of hyperthermia, bleomycin and X-rays on Ehrlich ascites tumor. J Surg Res 41:503–509
2. Matsuoka H, Sugimachi K, Mori M, Kuwano H, Ohno S, Nakano S (1989) Effects of hyperthermochemoradiotherapy on KSE-1 cells, a newly established human squamous cell line derived from esophageal carcinoma. Eur Surg Res 2:49–59
3. Crile G (1963) The effects of heat and radiation on cancers implanted on the feet of mice. Cancer Res 23:372–380
4. Hahn GM (1979) Potential for therapy of drugs and hyperthermia. Cancer Res 39:2264–2268
5. Suit HD, Gerweck LE (1979) Potential for hyperthermia and radiation therapy. Cancer Res 39:2290–2298
6. Ben-Hur E, Elkind MM, Bronk BV (1974) Thermally enhanced radioresponse of cultured Chinese hamster cells. Radiat Res 58:38–51
7. Stewart FA, Denekamp J (1978) The therapeutic advantage of combined heat and X rays on a mouse fibrosarcoma. Br J Radiol 51:307–316
8. Overgaad J (1980) Simultaneous and sequential hyperthermia and radiation treatment of an experimental tumor and its surrounding tissue in vivo. Int J Radiat Oncol Biol Phys 6:1507–1517
9. Marmor JB, Kozak D, Hahn GM (1979) Effects of systemically administered bleomycin or adriamycin with local hyperthermia on primary tumor and lung metastases. Cancer Treat Rep 63:1279–1290
10. Leith JT, Miller RC, Gerner EW, Boone LM (1977) Hyperthermic potentiation – biological aspects and applications to radiation therapy. Cancer 39:766–779
11. Braun J, Hahn GM (1975) Enhanced cell killing by bleomycin and 43 °C hyperthermia and the inhibition of recovery from potentially lethal damage. Cancer Res 35:2921–2927
12. Matsuoka H, Sugimchi K, Ueo H, Kuwano H, Nakano S, Nakayama M (1987) Sex hormone response of a newly established squamous cell line derived from clinical esophageal carcinoma. Cancer Res 47:4134–4140
13. Thomlinson RH, Gray LH (1955) The histological structure of some human lung cancers and the possible implications for radiotherapy. Br J Cancer 9:539–549

14. Manning MR, Cetas TC, Miller RC, Oleason JR, Connor WG, Gerner EW (1982) Clinical hyperthermia – results of a phase 1 trial employing hyperthermia alone or in combination with external beam or interstitial radiotherapy. Cancer 49:205–216
15. Sugimachi K, Inokuchi K, Kai H, Kuwano H, Matsuzaki K, Okudaira Y (1983) Hyperthermo-chemo-radiotherapy for carcinoma of the esophagus. Jpn J Surg 13:101–105
16. Hand JW (1987) Heat delivery and thermometry in clinical hyperthermia. In: Streffer C (ed) Recent results in cancer research. Springer, Berlin Heidelberg New York, pp 1–23
17. Dickson JA, Shah SA (1977) Technology for the hyperthermic treatment of large solid tumors at 50°C. Clin Oncol 3:301–318
18. Kim JH, Hahn EW, Tokita N, Nisce LZ (1977) Local tumor hyperthermia in combination with radiation therapy. Cancer 40:161–169
19. Leveen H, Wapnic S, Piccone V, Falk G, Ahmed N (1976) Tumor eradication by radiofrequency therapy. Response in 21 patients. JAMA 235:2198–2200
20. Marmor JB, Pounds D, Hahn GM (1987) Clinical trial of ultrasound induced hyperthermia. Proc 14th annual Meeting of the American Society of Clinical Oncology 19, p 330
21. Stehlin JS, Giovanella BC, Ipolyi PD, Muenz LR, Anderson RF (1975) Results of hyperthermic perfusion for melanoma of the extremities. Surg Gynecol Obstet 140:339–348
22. Qui SL, Li DJ, Shao LF, Wang CQ (1982) A pathological study on intraluminal microwave hyperthermia in esophageal cancer. NCI Monogr 61:415–417
23. Sugimachi K, Inokuchi K, Kai H, Sogawa A, Kawai Y (1983) Endotract antenna for application of hyperthermia to malignant lesions. Gann 74: 622–624
24. Sugaar S, Leveen HH (1979) A histopathologic study on the effects of radiofrequency thermotherapy on malignant tumors of the lung. Cancer 43:767–783
25. Sugimachi K, Kai H, Matsufuji H, Ueo H, Inokuchi K (1986) Histopathological evaluation of hyperthermo-chemo-radiotherapy for carcinoma of the esophagus. J Surg Oncol 32:82–85
26. Japanese Society of Esophageal Diseases (1976) Guidelines for the clinical and pathological studies for carcinoma of the esophagus. Jpn J Surg 6:79–86
27. Sugimachi K, Yaita A, Ueo H, Natsuda Y, Inokuchi K (1980) A safer and more reliable operative technique for esophageal reconstruction using a gastric tube. Am J Surg 140:471–474
28. Sugimachi K, Matsufuji H, Kai H, Matsuda H, Ueo H, Inokuchi K, Jingu K (1986) Preoperative irradiation for carcinoma of the esophagus. Surg Gynecol Obstet 162: 174–176
29. Koyama Y (1981) I-Hexylcarbamoyl-5-fluorouracil (HCFU) masked 5-fluorinated pyrimidine. Cancer Treat Rev 8:147–156
30. Iizuka T, Endo M, Sasaki K, Karasawa K, Kakegawa T, Arimori M, Sasaki T (1980) Preliminary report on multidisciplinary treatment for esophageal carcinoma. Jpn J Clin Oncol 10:215–220
31. Mondovi B, Strom R, Rotilio G, Finazzi Agro A, Cavaliele R, Rossi Fanelli A (1969) The biochemical mechanism of selective heat sensitivity of cancer cells – I. Studies on cellular respiration. Eur J Cancer 5:129–136
32. Mondovi B, Finazzi Agro A, Rotilio G, Strom R, Moricca G, Rossi Fanelli A (1969) The biochemical mechanism of selective heat sensitivity of cancer cells – II. Studies on nucleic acids and protein synthesis. Eur J Cancer 5:137–146
33. Chen TT, Heidelberger C (1969) Quantitative studies on the malignant transformation of mouse prostate cells by carcinogenic hydrocarbons in vitro. Int J Cancer 4:166–178
34. Giovanella BC, Morgan AC, Stehlin JS, Williams LJ (1973) Selective lethal effect of supranormal temperatures on mouse sarcoma cells. Cancer Res 33:2568–2578
35. Kase K, Hahn GM (1975) Differential heat response of normal and transformed human cells in tissue culture. Nature 255:228–230
36. Maehara Y, Kusumoto T, Kusumoto H, Anai H, Akazawa K, Sugimachi K (1988) Excised human neoplastic tissues are more sensitive to heat than the adjacent normal tissues. Eur Surg Res 20:254–259
37. Maehara Y, Anai H, Tamada R, Sugimachi K (1986) Partial hepatectomy alters sensitivity of rat hepatocytes to 5-fluorouracil. Cancer Lett 31:227–233
38. Maehara Y, Anai H, Sugimachi K (1987) Poorly differentiated human gastric carcinoma is more sensitive to antitumor drugs than is well differentiated carcinoma. Eur J Surg Oncol 13:203–206
39. Sugimachi K, Inokuchi K, Kai H, Ueo H, Kuwano H, Matsufuji H (1984) Preoperative hyperthermo-chemo-radiotherapy effective for carcinoma of the esophagus. J Surg Oncol 27:199–204
40. Hiraoka M, Jo S, Dodo Y, Ono K, Takahashi M, Nishida H, Abe M (1984) Clinical results of radiofrequency hyperthermia combined with radiation in the treatment of radioresistant cancers. Cancer 54: 2898–2904
41. Mosmann T (1983) Rapid colorimetric assay for cellular growth and survival: application to proliferation and cytotoxicity assays. J Immunol Methods 65:55–63
42. Cole SPC (1986) Rapid chemosensitivity testing of human lung tumor cells using the MTT assay. Cancer Chemother Pharmacol 17:259–263
43. Anai H, Maehara Y, Kusumoto H, Sugimachi K (1987) Comparison of the chemosensitivity of human neoplastic tissues between succinate dehydrogenase inhibition test and ATP assay. Clin Chim Acta 166:107–109
44. Anai H, Maehara Y, Kusumoto H, Sugimachi K (1987) Comparison between succinate dehydrogenase inhibition test and subrenal capsula assay for chemosensitivity testing. Oncology 44:115–117
45. Roti Roti JL (1982) Heat-induced cell death and radiosensitization: molecular mechanism. NC Monogr 61:3–10
46. Streffer C (1982) Aspects of biochemical effects by hyperthermia. NCI Monogr 61:11–17
47. Weber G (1977) Enzymology of cancer cells. N Engl J Med 296:486–493
48. Maehara Y, Nakamura H, Nakane Y, Kawai K, Okamoto M, Nagayama S, Shirasaka T, Fujii S (1982) Activities of various enzymes of pyrimidine nucleotide and DNA syntheses in normal and neoplastic human tissue. Gann 73:289–298

4 Combined Hyperthermia and Chemotherapy for Malignant Melanoma of the Limbs

F. Truchetet, E. Grosshans, J.C. Kretz, J. Friedel, and C. Chartier

4.1 Concepts and Problems in the Treatment of Malignant Melanomas

Malignant melanoma represents about 5% of skin cancers and 2% of malignant tumors (excluding the other skin cancers). Its incidence is extremely variable and is evaluated at 0.3/100000 inhabitants in Japan and up to 40/100000 inhabitants in Queensland, Australia, a number which is considered the highest in the world.

All the epidemiological studies stress that the incidence has varied in time and that it has increased dramatically during the last four decades. The incidence has roughly doubled over a period of 10 years in the countries where malignant melanomas are most frequent (Australia, United States, Scandinavia). This increased frequency is limited to certain ethnic groups and mostly concerns white populations with a fair phototype. In comparison to this latter group, the incidence is 6- to 15-fold less in blacks and the dark-skinned Caucasoid population.

The origin of malignant melanoma is multifactorial and, among the factors which influence its genesis, an important element is sunlight and its ultraviolet rays. Short, massive, and repeated exposures to sunlight which are characteristic of leisure activities clearly have the most harmful effects.

Four groups of malignant melanoma can be distinguished:

1. Superficial spreading melanoma is the most frequent type and represents 50% – 70% of cases; this malignant melanoma appears as a flat or slightly raised patch with a slow superficial horizontal extension which develops over several months before developing a vertical nodular extension.
2. Nodular melanoma constitutes 10% – 20% of cases and appears as a biologically aggressive tumor with immediate invasive and evolutionary potential.
3. Lentigo malignant melanoma develops on a preliminary lentigo maligna (LM) and represents 5% – 15% of cases; LM is an in situ melanoma which develops in patients aged more than 60 and most often on the face. This precancerous melanosis has a very prolonged horizontal evolution which may last for 5 – 20 years and its transformation into a malignant invasive melanoma only happens after a very prolonged interval.
4. Acrolentiginous melanoma constitutes 5% – 10% of cases and is most frequent in blacks and dark skinned Caucasoids; this malignant melanoma has a radial growth followed by a vertical growth and is most prominently situated on palms and soles and on digits.

These four clinical groups each have different histopathological characteristics which allow them to be distinguished from each other. Histopathology also permits the definition of histoprognostic indexes. These indexes make it possible to establish a correlation between the length of survival and the level of invasion. Presently, they also influence therapeutic decisions and guide the width of the excision margin. Clark's index represents the level of invasion:

Level I: the process is strictly limited to the epidermis (melanoma in situ)
Level II: malignant cells are detected in the papillary dermis
Level III: tumoral cells invade all the papillary dermis
Level IV: the reticular dermis is invaded
Level V: the fatty subcutis is invaded.

A poorer prognosis is correlated with a more invasive tumor. This invasion index is backed up by a second parameter, i.e., the thickness of the lesion according to Breslow's index (Fig. 4.1), which is in fact the most reliable prognostic index.

Such are the epidemiological, clinical, and histological characteristics of malignant melanomas which appear in the leading group of the most fearsome cancers. Incidence steadily grows and prognosis remains very poor. Although drastic therapeutic progress is still lacking, the treatment strategy for malignant melanoma has changed in recent decades because of a

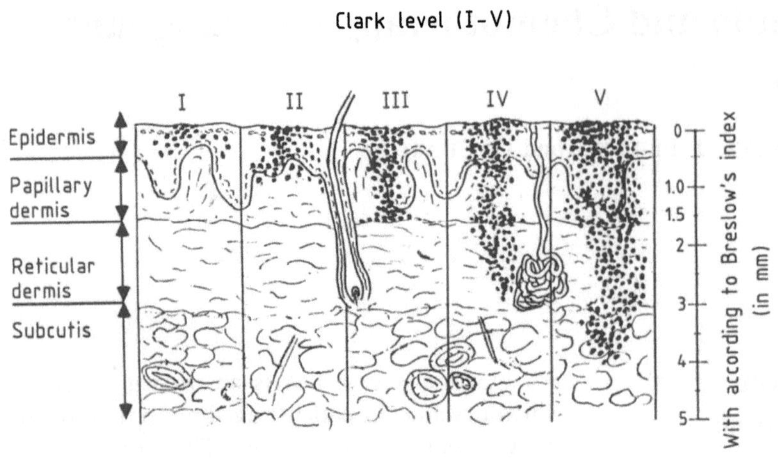

Fig. 4.1. Histoprognostic indexes according to Clark and Breslow

better understanding of the tumoral process and thanks to therapeutic protocols established and randomized among associated medical teams.

Surgery is unquestionably the treatment of choice and must be applied at the earliest possible stage of the illness. This surgery is guided by the preliminary histopathological examination. Prophylaxis appears as a fundamental necessity and the optimal situation would combine both preventive measures and the earliest possible detection and excision. Adjuvant therapeutic measures, either chemotherapeutic or immunotherapeutic, are destined to complete the effect of the initial treatment, but until now have not been proven to have any effect on the global survival rate and the number of recurrences.

In the metastatic disease, chemotherapy, hormonotherapy, radiotherapy, and the use of biological response modifiers are disappointing, and this relative therapeutic ineffectiveness is the main reason for the multiplication of other proposed measures. Among these measures, regional thermochemotherapy, used as a complement for surgery, appears as a novel technique. Although it was described more than three decades ago and its results are much debated, this technique appears to be beneficial in more than one situation.

4.2 Biological Basis of Combined Hyperthermia and Chemotherapy

The concept and technique of regional chemotherapy using intraarterial infusion of a cytotoxic drug was proposed in 1950 by Klopp et al. [22]. All the details were then settled, and the technique itself (including an extracorporeal circulation device) was introduced into clinical use for the first time in 1957, by Creech et al. [6]. This method of treatment appeared particularly interesting mainly because it allowed high doses of a drug to be brought to a precise region, at the same time avoiding their systemic toxic side-effects. Drug doses were only limited by the local tolerance capacity of tissues. This therapeutic means has been used in the treatment of different types of tumor and in most regions of the human body, and the best results have been registered with malignant melanomas of the limbs. A decade passed and in 1967 Stehlin [42], impressed by the works of Cavaliere et al. [5], proposed the association of hyperthermia with the regional chemotherapy device, stressing the importance of a synergistic effect of both hyperthermia and chemotherapy. This synergy may be explained by more than one mechanism [6, 20, 23, 45]:

1. Increased membrane permeability caused by elevated temperatures, allowing a better intracellular penetration of the chemical agent
2. Thermal inhibition of the repair procedures of the potentially lethal lesions induced by the cytotoxic drug
3. Enhancement of an antitumoral immune reaction by the liberation of tumoral antigenic substances during the cellular destruction phase which is induced by the associated chemotherapy and hyperthermia
4. Higher thermosensitivity of neoplastic cells as compared to normal cells, especially in the particular conditions induced by the extracorporeal circulation: chronic hypoxemia, nutritional deprivation, and tissular acidification.

The most frequently used drug is melphalan, according to Luck [30]. A retrospective study by Stehlin et al. in 1975 [43] showed that, among 165 patients, impressive results could be obtained in the treatment of malignant melanomas with satellite metastases, with a 300% amelioration of the survival rate (22%–77%).

Regional thermochemotherapy has subsequently been regularly used and has yielded variable and debatable results in the treatment of malignant melanomas of the limbs [37, 38]. Indications are limited to primary malignant melanomas with high evolutive risk. This risk is evaluated according to Clark's level and Breslow's index; the tumors which are considered as leading to a high risk are primary malignant melanomas with a Clark level of III or more and a Breslow index equal to, or higher than, 1.5 mm. This method of treatment is also reserved for malignant melanomas of the limbs with regional metastatic dissemination (satellite, in transit, or lymph node metastases). During recent years, technical progress has permitted an optimization of the therapeutic results together with a lessening of the complications [27].

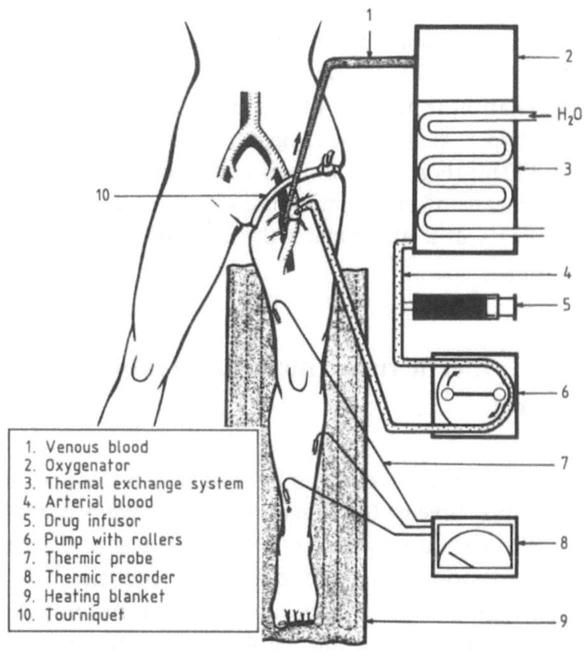

Fig. 4.2. Diagram of the extracorporeal circulation device allowing performance of a regional hyperthermic perfusion of melphalan before surgical removal of the melanoma

4.3 Treatment Techniques and Protocols
[23, 37, 39]

4.3.1 Extracorporeal Circulation

The surgical operation is conducted under general anesthesia. The surgical site is proximal: for the upper limbs access is most often axillary, and less frequently subclavicular; for the lower limbs access may be iliac, femoral, or popliteal.
An external iliac access is essentially used for lesions situated on the higher portion of the thigh or for cases with inguinal metastatic lymph nodes. This access allows easier lymph node evacuation and the postoperative edema is much less important in this case.
Heparinization is then induced (3 mg/kg or 150 U/kg body weight). Krementz and co-workers stress the fact that heparin probably has an antimetastatic effect by means of an inhibiting action on the tumoral cell adhesion on the vascular walls [23, 27]. Heparin could also have a specific tumoricidal effect [35].
Once heparinization has been induced, cannulae are placed into the vascular channels and are connected to an extracorporeal circulation device (Fig. 4.2) which includes an oxygenator, a thermal exchange system, and a pump. Blood escape via the collateral circulation towards the general circulation is prevented by placing a tourniquet above the vascular access. Most authors recommend the use of a colored tracer such as Evans blue or fluorescein or even radioactive tracer such as ^{131}I-labeled albumin for the detection of escaping blood. Perfusion is interrupted if such escape corresponds to more than 10%–15% of the total dose. We personally do not use these tracers and follow Cruchley et al. [7], who evaluate the escape according to the level of the blood in the oxygenator, a steady level being the indication of an isolated blood circulation. This method is not totally reliable as the level may remain steady with equivalent double direction escape. Most studies point out that escape may be considered minimal if the perfusion pressure remains lower than the diastolic systemic arterial pressure by 10–20 mmHg [13, 23]. Moreover, Fontijne et al. have shown that an optimal tissue perfusion may be obtained when the pressure gradient between the systemic arterial blood and the blood in the limb does not exceed 15 mmHg [13]. Ghussen et al. have evaluated the blood escape to be less than 10% in 95% of perfusion cases and to be between 10% and 20% in 5% of cases when the perfusion pressure stays around 80 mmHg [14].
The extracorporeal circulation is then initiated, including an overheating of the limb caused by heating the perfusion liquid when it passes through the heat exchange device. Some authors recommend the use of a sterile blanket placed around the perfused limb, including a water circuit to maintain the proper temperature and avoid thermal losses.
The infusion flow varies from 0.5 to 1.5 liter/min and depends on the diameter of the blood vessels and of

the cannulae. High flows permit a better tissular perfusion and lessen the toxicity, and also accelerate the heating of the limb to the desired tissular temperature. Oxygenation in the circuit is most often described as being hyperoxemic with oxygen pressures between 300 and 400 mmHg. High oxygen concentrations are another means of potentiating the effects of the alkylating agents and also have a direct tumoricidal effect [10, 24].

4.3.2 Hyperthermia (Including Temperature Control)

Temperatures are measured by means of a thermal recorder via three or four thermal probes. We personally use three probes leading to the peritumoral tissues, to the hypodermic tissues, and to the muscles.
The infusion of the drug is induced when the temperature reaches 38 °C. Our choice has gone towards melphalan and we distribute the total dose in three boluses at 3-min intervals, directly in the artery as suggested by Krementz et al. [27]. Others have proposed a single infusion of the total dose in the pump reservoir [27]. The tissular temperature is then maintained between 40° and 41.5 °C for between 45 min and 1 h, depending on the authors.
Extracorporeal circulation is then interrupted and the limb is drained of its blood before the tourniquet is removed so as to avoid the passage of an important quantity of the drug to the general circulation. Most authors describe the use of 500–1000 ml dextran and then of 250–500 ml blood. When the cannulae have been withdrawn, the heparinization is compensated by protamine sulfate. The incisions are then stitched up and finally the tumor (or the excision scar) is excised with a margin of 3 cm.
Postoperatively, effective anticoagulation is maintained for 6 weeks.

4.3.3 Chemotherapy

Melphalan is the most frequently used drug. This *p*-di-(2-chloroethyl)amino-L-phenylalanine is derived from phenylalanine and shares its metabolic destiny especially in the melanocyte. It acts as an alkylating agent and is derived from mechlorethamine, a nitrosourea mustard. Doses are 1–1.5 mg/kg body weight for a lower limb and 0.5–1 mg/kg body weight for an upper limb.
Some authors are in favor of an adapted dosage according to the volume of the perfused limb [50, 52]. The optimal dosage is estimated at 10 mg/liter of perfused tissue, the volume of the limb being the displaced water volume when the limb is immersed in a bath.
Krementz et al. have compared the two means of evaluating the dosage [46]: for an upper limb the dose is cut by 45% when the dosage is estimated by the volume technique, as opposed to the body weight technique; for a lower limb the dose is raised by 15% with the volume technique. Recent recommendations for the estimation of doses according to the volume speak of 10 mg/liter for lower limbs and 13 mg/liter for upper limbs [27]. Whatever method is used, the proposed concentrations of drug in the perfused parts are six- to ten-fold those obtained with classic systemic infusions [20, 23].
In some studies on hyperthermia, drug concentrations in the blood, measured by high performance liquid chromatography, are evaluated between 6.1 to 115 μg/ml, which represents a 10- to 100-fold higher concentration than that obtained with classic intravenous infusions [36].
Concentrations of melphalan in the perfusion liquid quickly drop (in less than an hour) in all patients.
Catabolites are mainly represented by:

1. Monohydroxymelphalan with its highest concentration after about 1 h and 45 min; it disappears after 6 h
2. Dihydroxymelphalan with its highest concentration after 1 h; it disappears 4 h after infusion.

These catabolites are eliminated through the urine. Thus melphalan is the object of a quick hydrolyzation which inactivates its action. Melphalan is also quickly captured by the perfused tissues, a mechanism which is saturated after 30 min. The half-life of the drug is shortened by this tissular capture and also by a capture in the filters and the extracorporeal circulation piping.
Hydrolysis is dependent on many factors such as:

1. The temperature: when it is higher than 42 °C, the alkylating agents are more quickly hydrolyzed and the toxicity is worsened
2. The pH
3. The type of perfusion liquid.

Other drugs have been used alone or in association [2, 3, 11, 21, 41] with the following dosages according to the volume of the limb:

Dacarbazine 100 mg/liter
Cisplatinum 15–20 mg/liter
D-Actinomycin 0.1 mg/liter
Vindesine 0.3 to 0.4 mg/liter.

In a study by Martijn et al. the association of D-actinomycin and melphalan did not yield better results than melphalan alone [31].
Thus technical operative progress and a better knowledge of the pharmacology of the used drugs have been the conditions for and means of obtaining better therapeutic results together with an appreciable lessening of side-effects.

4.4 Clinical Trials and Results: The Strasbourg Experience

4.4.1 Technical Characteristics, Selection Criteria, and Exclusion Criteria

In our experience, the femoral pathway was exclusively used for the treatment on the lower limbs and the axillary pathway for treatment on the upper limbs. Melphalan was the only drug which was used, and doses were 1.4 mg/kg body weight for lower limbs and 0.9 mg/kg body weight for upper limbs. Perfusion under hyperthermia was maintained for 45 min and we never carried out any kind of prophylactic lymph node evacuation.

Selection Criteria. Until 1984, this regional thermochemotherapy was used for the treatment of malignant melanomas of the limbs with a Breslow index higher than 0.85 mm. After 1984 the technique was only applied to malignant melanomas with a Breslow index equal to or higher than 1.5 mm. The localization had to be within the following limits:

1. Under the level of insertion of the deltoid muscle on the arm for the upper limbs
2. Under the lower level of the upper third of the thigh for the lower limbs.

Exclusion Criteria. These were limited to possible alterations of the main vascular channels such as arteriopathy and thrombophlebitis.
Cases were categorized under the classification used by the M.D. Anderson Hospital:

Stage I: primary malignant melanomas only
Stage II: recurrences or satellite lesions when limited within a local radius of 3 cm
Stage III: regional metastases
A: either in transit
B: or concerning lymph nodes
AB (or C): or both in transit and in lymph nodes
Stage IV: distant metastases.

Between January 1982 and January 1987, 68 patients with malignant melanomas of the limbs were thus proposed for this protocol with associated surgical excision of their lesion. Five patients were excluded from the study for technical reasons such as too small a caliber of the main blood vessels which would not have allowed a sufficient flow. We would like to stress that these were five women, each with a malignant melanoma situated on an upper limb.

4.4.2 Complications and Side-effects

A classification of complications of thermochemotherapy for malignant melanomas under extracorporeal circulation has been proposed by Wieberdink et al. and comprises five stages [22, 52]:

Stage I: absence of reaction
Stage II: inconspicuous erythema and/or edema
Stage III: noticeable erythema and edema, possibly with blisters
Stage IV: large blistering dermatosis and deep tissular alterations with prominent functional impotence
Stage V: severe reaction leading to amputation.

These locoregional complications may be complemented by the existence of medullary depression with leukopenia, the acme of which occurs around the 12th postoperative day.
In our series, the postoperative period was most often free of important side-effects, and when these occurred they always regressed spontaneously. General side-effects were limited to:

1. Digestive embarrassment such as nausea and vomiting, sometimes for 3 days running
2. Cytopenia with:
   a) Constant anemia due partly to hemodilution and partly to the passage of melphalan in the general circulation
   b) Frequent transitory leukopenia
   c) Temporary thrombopenia (only one case was observed)

All of these cytopenic accidents happened during the first 4 postoperative weeks and regressed spontaneously.
Locoregional side-effects were:

1. Mild erythema and/or edema constantly. Edema may be prevented by a systematically placed elastic bandage, the wearing of which we advise for the first 3 months

2. A discrete functional impotence of the treated limb was often observed and justified early reeducation, so as to avoid ankylosis and retraction of tendons. One patient experienced severe trophic alterations with large blisters, dysesthesia, and temporary ankylosis (stage IV).

Miscellaneous complications were:

1. A case of arterial wounding
2. A case of early postoperative thrombophlebitis.

Lastly, we sometimes observed side-effects without serious consequences such as:

1. A mild postedemic skin desquamation
2. Sudden interruption of the growth of nails with their ultimate shedding on the treated limb.

Thus, mortality was nonexistent and morbidity was low in our series. Reviewing the literature, and adding up the results of 2500 perfusions reported in the literature, we can see a global mortality due to this type of surgery of about 1% of cases; among the most serious complications are the necessity for an amputation in 0.7% of cases and a loss of the function of the limb in another 3%. It is to be observed that with the passage of time and the development of more experienced teams, the complications of this technique are becoming much less frequent (Table 4.1).

4.4.3 Results

In the period from January 1982 to January 1987, we regularly followed up 63 patients who underwent surgery with regional thermochemotherapy for a malignant melanoma of a limb. Among these were 14 men (22%) and 49 women (78%). Mean age was 50.5 years (51 years for women and 47 years for men), with extremes of 23 and 74 years.

The primary tumor was on an upper limb in 17 cases (27%) and on a lower limb in 46 cases (73%). This predominance of cases on lower limbs is due to the predominance of women in our series, as women preferentially have malignant melanomas on their lower limbs.

Histological types were distributed as follows:

1. Superficial spreading melanoma	19 (30%)
2. Nodular melanoma	24 (38%)
3. Acrolentiginous melanoma	17 (27%)
4. Unspecified type of melanoma	3 (5%)

The patient groups according to the M.D. Anderson Hospital classification were distributed as follows:

Stage I		49 (78%)
Stage II		7 (11%)
Stage III	A	5 (8%)
	B	1 (1.5%)
	AB(C)	1 (1.5%)
Stage IV		0

During the 5-year follow-up, seven patients (11%) died of metastatic extensions of the disease. Among these, three were classified in the stage I group, and all had lesions with a Breslow index higher than 1.5 mm, one was classified in the stage II group at inclusion, and three were classified in the stage III group at inclusion. Their overall mean survival was 13.5 months.

January 1987 saw 56 living patients (89%). Four patients were found to have locoregional recurrences, either satellites or in transit or in lymph nodes (6.5%); one patient was found to have systemic metastases (1.5%); and 51 patients were apparently free of all metastatic extensions (81%).

Thus, the actuarial survival rate after 5 years is 79.5% if one takes all stages into consideration. It is 85.5% for the stage I group and 81.8% if one considers a Breslow index equal to or higher than 1.5 mm (Fig. 4.3). Our results are comparable to those in the literature, where the survival rate after 5 years is reported to be between 79% and 86% [8, 27].

The actuarial survival rate is 83% for the stage II group, but it can only be calculated on the basis of a period of 39 months; it is 41.5% for the stage III group based on a period of only 15 months. The inadequate number of patients in these two groups and moreover the insufficient length of observation do not allow interpretation of the results for stage II and III patients (Fig. 4.4).

More than one author stresses the influence of the localization of the malignant melanoma on the therapeutic result. In our series the survival rate after 5

Table 4.1. Series with hyperthermic perfusions and evaluation of complications

Authors	Date of publication	Number of cases
Shingleton et al. [40]	1975	43
McBride et al. [34]	1975	244
Stehlin et al. [43]	1975	185
Sugarbaker and McBride [46]	1976	213
Wagner [51]	1976	245
Bulman and Jamieson [4]	1980	70
Ghussen et al. [14]	1981	87
Janoff et al. [20]	1982	122
Tonak et al. [49]	1984	251
Schraffordt-Koops et al. [39]	1985	152
Krementz et al. [27]	1987	897

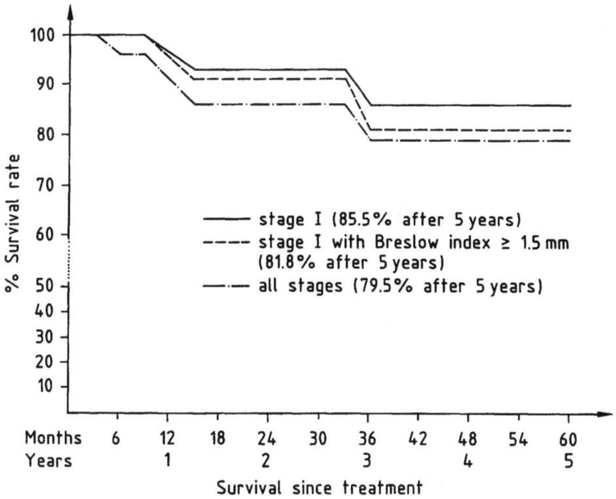

Fig. 4.3. Five-year actuarial rates of cases of malignant melanoma included under the regional extracorporeal thermochemotherapy protocol. Total number of patients: 63; stage I (primary tumor without recurrence or metastasis): 49 cases; stage I with Breslow index equal to or higher than 1.5 mm: 37 cases

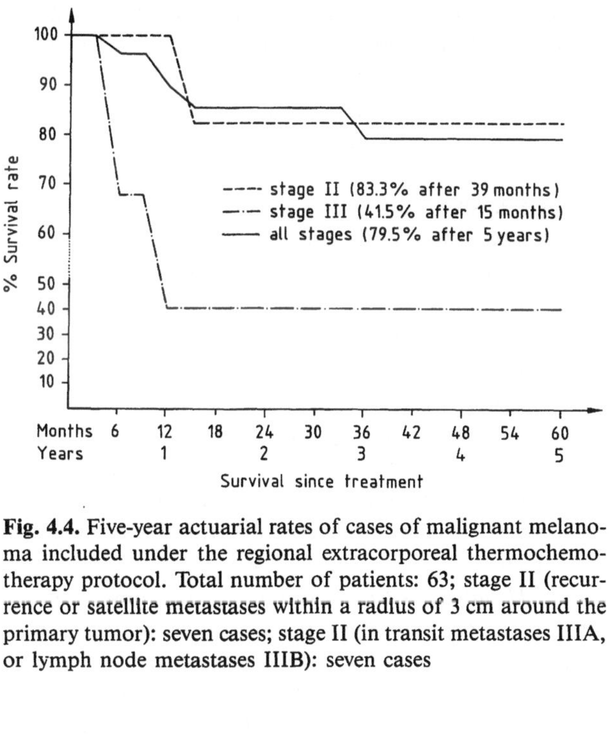

Fig. 4.4. Five-year actuarial rates of cases of malignant melanoma included under the regional extracorporeal thermochemotherapy protocol. Total number of patients: 63; stage II (recurrence or satellite metastases within a radius of 3 cm around the primary tumor): seven cases; stage II (in transit metastases IIIA, or lymph node metastases IIIB): seven cases

years is 100% in patients with malignant melanomas of the upper limbs whereas it is 70.7% in patients with malignant melanomas of the lower limbs. These results, which are similar to those published by Krementz et al. [27], must be contrasted with those published by Schraffordt-Koops et al. [39], who report a better survival rate with malignant melanomas of the lower limbs. As a matter of fact when results are subgrouped according to sex and localization, it appears that the survival rate is the same with upper limbs and lower limbs in women, whereas according to Krementz et al. in men the survival rate is better for upper limb localizations [27].

The 5-year survival rate in the stage I patients is 82% for malignant melanomas of the upper limbs and 69% for malignant melanomas of the lower limbs. Schraffordt-Koops et al. [39] and Krementz et al. [27] also consider that the result is influenced by the localization of the malignant melanoma on the limb. Hand and foot malignant melanomas are less sensitive to treatment than proximally situated malignant melanomas. Krementz et al. [27] report 10-years survival rates of 62% and 61% for hand and foot malignant melanomas respectively and of 89% and 85% for malignant melanomas of the thighs and arms. These authors consider the plantar and subungual localizations to carry the worst prognostic significance, with a 10-year survival rate of 41%. In a retrospective comparison of surgery alone versus thermochemotherapy combined with surgery for stage I malignant melanomas of the limbs with a Breslow index higher than 1.5 mm, Martijn et al. [33] report an obviously more beneficial effect of thermochemotherapy for malignant melanomas situated on the lower limbs and for lesions situated on the legs: in this case the 10-year survival rate is 80.8%, against 60.3% with surgery alone. In contrast there appears to be no significant amelioration of the survival rate for malignant melanomas situated on the foot: the 10-year survival rate is 53.4% for surgery plus thermochemotherapy and 50.3% for surgery alone. Thus a beneficial effect of the hyperthermic perfusion appears dubious to these authors as far as lesions of the foot are concerned.

In a retrospective study, Fletcher et al. [12] are in disagreement with these last results as they report a 5-year survival rate of 75% for acrolentiginous melanoma stages I and II when treated with surgery plus regional thermochemotherapy. These authors compare their results with those of the literature, which report the 5-year survival rate after conventional surgery for acrolentiginous melanoma as being between 30% and 43%.

4.5 Discussion and Comments

Our results are an illustration of all the present controversies which are to be found in the literature.

The main criticism leveled at the supporters of the thermochemotherapy technique concerns the absence of any randomized prospective study which would make it possible to ascertain an objective superiority of surgery combined with hyperthermic perfusion

Table 4.2. Regional hyperthermic perfusion plus surgery for stage I malignant melanomas of the limbs: 5-year survival rates

Authors	Date of publication	5-year survival rates
Schraffordt-Koops et al. [39]	1985	79%
Krementz et al. [27]	1987	84%
Sugarbaker and McBride [46]	1976	88%
Davis et al. [9]	1976	90%
Wagner [51]	1976	93%
Martijn et al. [32]	1983	95%
Golomb et al. [18]	1979	96%

Table 4.3. Results of surgery for stage I malignant melanomas: 5-year survival rates according to literature from 1969 to 1979

Authors	Date of publication	5-year survival rates
Coppelant (cited in [34])	1969	51%
Knutson (cited in [26])	1971	58%
Tonak et al. [48]	1979	60%
Ariel (cited in [49])	1974	66%
Weidner (cited in [49])	1974	69%
Sugarbaker and McBride [46]	1976	70%
Bowden (cited in [26])	1976	71%

over surgery alone [23, 27, 36, 38, 39]: most of the published work is retrospective.

Comparison of the results of the different works which speak of the treatment of malignant melanomas by regional perfusion is made difficult by many factors which modify or influence the prognosis and which may introduce a bias, e.g., age, sex, localization, histological type, invasion level, effective state of the draining lymph node chains, other associated treatments, and variations in the modalities of the hyperthermic perfusion. Randomized studies initially seemed unnecessary after the first published results in the 1960s and 1970s [27].

4.5.1 Present Indications and Summary of Clinical Data

For stage I malignant melanoma, the 5-year survival rates appear to be between 79% and 96% (Table 4.2) and our results, reporting 85.5%, appear compatible with these figures. These results immediately appeared better than those of conventional surgery: Ackerman and Del Regato had reported a 45% survival rate after 5 years in stage I malignant melanomas [1], and the main studies devoted to surgery alone in the 1970s reported survival rates of between 51% and 71% after 5 years (Table 4.3). Concerning the hyperthermic perfusion technique, the authors who advocated it progressively considered that their results topped those of classical surgery by 10%–20% in stage I malignant melanomas [20]. But recent results with conventional surgery for stage I malignant melanomas speak of 5-year survival rates between 79% and 95% [27]. Thus the beneficial effect of the hyperthermic perfusion technique no longer appears so evident in stage I malignant melanomas.

Hyperthermic perfusion is thought to bring another advantage, namely the prevention of locoregional recurrences (satellite, in transit, or lymph node metastases), with a frequency of only about 3% [27]. This figure is much lower than those of 18%–33% reported with surgery alone [8]. But Schraffordt-Koops et al. report the frequency of local recurrences to be 13% when the survey is prolonged to between 5 and 18 years [39]. They stress that these recurrences mainly occur after 5 years and they therefore put forward the idea that the hyperthermic perfusion technique essentially delays more than prevents local recurrences. To their mind, the observation period should last for at least 10 years.

In such a situation prospective randomized studies appear absolutely indispensable so as to compare the two methods, especially as regards stage I malignant melanomas [8, 27, 36, 38].

For stage II malignant melanomas, differences in survival rates as reported in retrospective studies are much more clear-cut: 5-year survival rates are 15%–19% with surgery alone and 39%–68% with surgery combined with hyperthermic perfusion (Table 4.4). Thus thermochemotherapy allows a doubled survival rate compared to classical surgical treatment in this group.

Stage III malignant melanomas, in the view of many authors, appear the best indication for hyperthermic perfusion, especially as regards stage IIIA. Before the development of this technique the 5-year survival rates varied between 15% and 40% [28]. Thermochemotherapy gives results rarying between 28% and 67% (Table 4.5).

Stehlin et al. [43] alone give a 5-year survival rate over 70%. Figures 4.5 and 4.6 show our results with the technique in a stage III case at an interval of 5 months.

Krementz [27] and Sutherland [47] show that in stages IIIB and IIIAB the survival rate is a proportional function of the number of metastatic lymph nodes. When one lymph node is positive the 10-year survival rate is 64% [27]. On the other hand when many

Table 4.4. Stage II malignant melanomas: 5-year survival rates after surgery alone and surgery combined with extracorporeal hyperthermic perfusion

Authors	Date of publication	5-year survival rates	
Ackerman and Del Regato [1]	1962	15%	Surgery alone
Bowden (cited in [25])	1960	19%	
Krementz and Ryan [25]	1972	39%	Surgery combined with hyperthermic perfusion
Krementz et al. [26]	1979	62%	
Krementz [23]	1986	68%	
Schraffordt-Koops et al. [39]	1985	42%	
McBride et al. [34]	1971	57%	
Wagner [51]	1976	68%	

Table 4.5. Stage III malignant melanomas of the limbs: 5-year survival rates after regional hyperthermic perfusion

Authors	Date of publication	5-year survival rates
Stage IIIA:		
Shingleton et al. [40]	1975	28%
Krementz [23]	1986	29%
Schraffordt-Koops et al. [39]	1985	50%
McBride (cited in [29])	1979	51%
Bulman and Jamieson [4]	1980	52%
Stehlin et al. [43]	1975	77%
Stage IIIB:		
Schraffordt-Koops et al. [39]	1985	46%
Krementz [23]	1986	52%
Tonak et al. [49]	1983	67%
Stage IIIAB:		
Krementz et al. [27]	1986	31%
Schraffordt-Koops et al. [39]	1985	40%

lymph nodes are found to be positive the 10-year survival rate only reaches 24% [27]. In some of these conditions thermochemotherapy may represent a palliative means of saving a limb [29]. These studies are nonetheless largely controversial and many other works, especially those of Storm and Morton, question the results [44]. These authors report an excellent local response in 21 out of 26 patients (81%) with stage II and III malignant melanomas of the lower limbs. This method of treatment may have a palliative significance but the overall mean survival rate after 3 years is less than 25%. They consider the technique to be excellent for locoregional control of the illness but of no significance as regards survival. We would nonetheless like to mention the encouraging randomized prospective study by Ghussen et al. [15], who reported results in 107 cases of malignant melanomas with Clark levels III, IV, and V and Breslow indexes

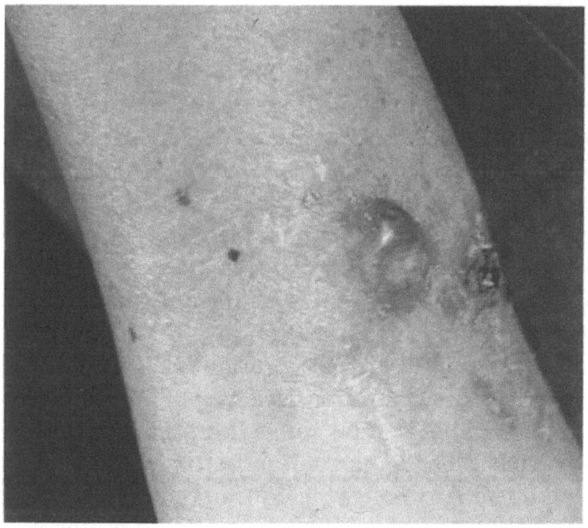

Fig. 4.5. Nodular melanoma of the left leg with in situ metastatic dissemination in a woman aged 50, before extracorporeal circulation thermochemotherapy

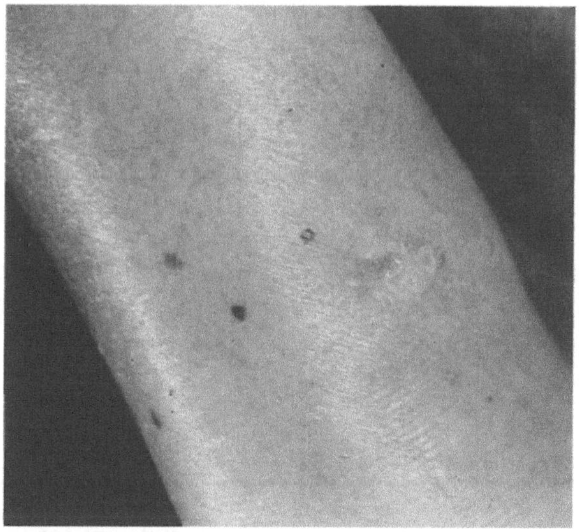

Fig. 4.6. Aspects of the left leg in the same patient as in Fig. 4.5, 5 months after thermochemotherapy. Note the persistent black tattoos which correspond to undigested melanin in the upper chorion in the places where metastases have been destroyed (histopathologically ascertained)

Table 4.6. Recurrence rates (%) in the two groups in Ghussen et al.'s study [15] (see text)

	Stage I	Stage II	Stage III
Group A	27.8%	31.6%	58.8%
Group B	5.6%	5.5%	12.5%

Table 4.7. Recurrence-free intervals[a] in the two groups in Ghussen et al.'s study [15] (see text)

	Stage I	Stage II	Stage III
Group A	174	115	195
Group B	540	488	708

[a] Delay of recurrence expressed in days

equal to or higher than 1.5 mm. Two groups were compared: in the first (A), 54 patients had conventional surgical treatment with prophylactic lymph node evacuation; in the second (B), 53 patients underwent regional thermochemotherapy with melphalan, combined with the same surgical treatment. The main criterion of efficacy was the recurrence-free interval over a mean time period of 550 days. Krementz stresses the fact that globally there is a maximum difference of 5% between the disease-free period and the overall survival time in patients with malignant melanomas [23]. The recurrence rate in the two groups was reported as significantly different (Table 4.6). Recurrence-free intervals were significantly longer in group B than in group A (Table 4.7).

These very important differences between the two techniques were so significant that randomization was considered indefensible by the authors from an ethical point of view. The results appeared significant enough to make the comparison of 5-year and 10-year survival rates seem unnecessary. A reevaluation of the results was performed 2 1/2 years later [16] and 3 1/2 years later [17, 18], and they still showed a very significantly favorable effect of the perfusion technique. These results, however, remain isolated in the world literature.

4.5.2 Future Prospects

Despite these encouraging results, indications for the perfusion technique should be proposed very cautiously because of the important investment as far as equipment, technical difficulty, financial cost, etc. is concerned. Results of other randomized studies should be awaited and should confirm these preliminary results before this therapeutic method is proposed as a routine treatment for high risk malignant melanomas of the limbs. Two such studies are underway under the aegis of the perfusionists' group of the European Organization for the Research and Treatment of Cancer (EORTC) and the North American Perfusion Group (NAPG).

4.6 Conclusion

In spite of more than 30 years' experience with the thermochemotherapy technique in some treatment centers, many uncertainties remain as regards indications for the perfusion, the proper drugs to be used and their posology, the role and importance of hyperthermia, and the true pharmacokinetics of the method. Controversy is also nourished by the fact that the failures are due to the systemic nature of the illness. Nonetheless, despite the global lack of randomized prospective studies, many authors who use thermochemotherapy for the treatment of malignant melanomas of the limbs consider that retrospective studies make it possible to say that the amelioration of the survival rates is from 10% to 20% with invasive malignant melanomas of the limbs when at stage I, compared to the rates with surgery alone. This difference in results should be verified by randomized prospective studies before drawing any sort of conclusion. In stage II and III malignant melanomas, results seem more clear-cut, and survival rates are doubled in some studies by the use of hyperthermic perfusion.

Lastly, in some advanced forms of the illness, isolated perfusions of a limb may offer an alternative to amputation or other major surgical decisions, as a means of ameliorating the quality of survival. Our study in Strasbourg can only be considered as preliminary because of the small patient numbers and the short observation times. Therefore, we retain a certain number of indications while waiting for the results of randomized prospective studies (EORTC, NAPG) and because of our results, which indicate some form of efficacy (a 5-year actuarial survival rate of 85.5% in stage I malignant melanomas with a Breslow index equal to or higher than 1.5 mm). This method, which is still experimental although described some decades ago, should be reserved for strictly established protocols so as to judge its true value. Our indications are: a) stage I malignant melanomas with a Breslow index equal to or higher than 1.5 mm; b) stage II and IIIA malignant melanomas.

In cases of stage II or III malignant melanoma, most authors recommend two perfusions separated by an interval of 6 weeks.

This complex technique, when in the hands of trained teams, provides a quantitative and qualitative amelioration of the survival together with very weak mortality and morbidity rates, which are acceptable in the presence of an illness with such a disastrous prognosis.

Future prospects as regards this technique seem quite open, and the large number of current studies should yield improved results together with:

1. A better understanding of the pharmacology of the drugs, with precise dosages and temperatures, optimal length of time for perfusion, etc.
2. Introduction of new drugs, possibly synergistic, such as alkylating agents and cisplatinum, or introduction of other therapeutic means such as associated radiotherapy [19]. The synergistic effect of hyperthermia and radiotherapy is presently the basis of a multicenter randomized study supervised by the European Society for Hyperthermic Oncology
3. Pretherapeutic evaluation of the tumoral specific sensitivity to various agents
4. Extension of the period of exposure of the tumor to a cytotoxic agent by means of the use of gel microspheres introduced in a targeted fashion into the circulation system of the tumor. The infusion of microspheres is then followed by a transitory thrombosis for 10–15 min, a means of augmenting the concentration of the drug in the vascular system of the tumor
5. Modification of the hyperthermic conditions with a more selective tumoral hyperthermia system
6. Use of monoclonal antibodies.

References

1. Ackerman LV, Del Regato JA (1962) Malignant melanoma of the skin. In: Cancer: diagnosis, treatment, and prognosis. Mosby -cV, St Louis
2. Aigner KR, Hild P, Hundeiker M (1981) Neue Entwicklungen in der isolierten Extremitäten Perfusion. Z Hautkr 57:1044–1054
3. Aigner KR, Walther H, Link KH, Voigt H (1986) Perfusionstherapie. In: Voigt H, Kleeber UR (eds) Malignes Melanom. Springer, Berlin Heidelberg New York, pp 299–305
4. Bulman AS, Jamieson CW (1980) Isolated limb perfusion with melphalan in the treatment of malignant melanoma. Br J Surg 67: 660–662
5. Cavaliere R, Ciocatto E, Giovanella B, Heidelberger C, Johnson R, Magottini M, Mondovi B, Moricca G, Rossi-Favelli A (1967) Selective heat sensitivity of cancer cells. Biochemical and clinical studies. Cancer 20:1351–1381
6. Creech O, Krementz ET, Ryan RF, Winblad JN (1958) Chemotherapy of cancer: regional perfusion utilizing an extracorporeal circuit. Ann Surg 148:616–632
7. Cruchley PM, Kaplan JA, Waller JL, Youg MR (1982) Anesthesia for isolated hyperthermic limb perfusion. Anesthesiology 57:228–230
8. Cumberlin R, De Moss E, Lassus M, Freidman M (1985) Isolation perfusion for malignant melanoma of the extremity: a review. J Clin Oncol 3:1022–1031
9. Davis CD, Ivins JC, Soule EH (1976) Mayo Clinic experience with isolated limb perfusion for invasive malignant melanoma of the extremities. Proceedings of the ninth international pigment cell conference, Houston Texas. In: Riley R (ed) Pigment cell. Karger S, New York, pp 379–385
10. De Cosse JJ, Rogers LS (1966) Influence of high pressure oxygen and chemotherapy of the A. Mel 4 hamster melanoma. Cancer Res pt 1:287–292
11. Didolkar MS, Fitzpatrick JL, Jackson AJ, Johnson GS (1986) Toxicity and complications of vascular isolation and hyperthermic perfusion with imidazole carboxamide in melanoma. Cancer 57:1961–1966
12. Fletcher JR, White CR, Fletcher WA (1986) Improved survival rates of patients with acral lentiginous melanoma treated with hyperthermic isolation perfusion, wide excision, and regional lymphadenectomy. Am J Surg 151:593–597
13. Fontijne WPJ, Mook PH, Schraffordt-Koops J, Oldhoff J, Wildevuur RH (1985) Improved tissue perfusion during pressure regulated hyperthermic regional isolated perfusion. A clinical study. Cancer 55:1455–1461
14. Ghussen F, Nagel K, Groth W (1981) Regionale hypertherme Zytostatikaperfusion bei malignen Melanomen der Extremitäten. Dtsch Med Wochenschr 106:1612–1615
15. Ghussen F, Nagel K, Groth W, Müller JM, Stützer H (1984) A prospective randomized study of regional extremity perfusion in patients with malignant melanoma. Ann Surg 200:764–768
16. Ghussen F, Kruger I, Groth W, Stützer H (1986) Randomized melanoma study of perfusion of the extremities. Results of treatment 2 1/2 years after premature discontinuation. Chirurg 57:619–623
17. Ghussen F, Kruger I, Groth W, Stützer H (1988) The role of regional hyperthermic cytostatic perfusion in the treatment of extremity melanoma. Cancer 61:654–659
18. Golomb FM, Bromberg J, Dubin N (1979) A controlled study of the survival experience of patients with primary malignant melanoma of the distal extremities treated with adjuvant isolated perfusion. Adjuvant Ther Cancer 2:519–526
19. Gundersen S, Hager B, Tausjø J (1986) Radiation in combination with intra-arterial infusion therapy with dacarbazine for metastatic malignant melanoma localized to a lower extremity. Cancer Treat Rev 70:1015–1017
20. Janoff KA, Moseson D, Nohlgren J, Davenport C, Richards C, Fletcher WS (1982) The treatment of stage I melanoma of the extremities with regional hyperthermic isolation perfusion. Ann Surg 196:316–323
21. Klein ES, Ben-Ari GY (1987) Isolation perfusion with cisplatin for malignant melanoma of the limbs. Cancer 59:1068–1071
22. Klopp C, Alford T, Bateman J, Berry G, Winship T (1950) Fractionated intra-arterial cancer chemotherapy with meth-

yl bis amine hydrochloride. A preliminary report. Ann Surg 132:811–832
23. Krementz ET (1986) Regional perfusion. Current sophistication, what next? Cancer 57:426–432
24. Krementz ET, Knudson L (1961) The effect of increased oxygen tension on the tumoricidal effect of nitrogen mustard. Surgery 50:266–271
25. Krementz ET, Ryan RF (1972) Chemotherapy of melanoma of the extremities by perfusion; fourteen years clinical experience. Ann Surg 175:900–917
26. Krementz ET, Carter RD, Sutherland CM, Campbell M (1979) The use of regional chemotherapy in the management of malignant melanoma. World J Surg 3:289–304
27. Krementz ET, Carter RD, Sutherland CM, Muchmore JH (1987) Chemotherapy by regional perfusion for limb melanoma. Am Surg 53:133–140
28. Lee YTNM (1980) Loco-regional recurrent melanoma. I. Natural history. Cancer Treat Rev 7:59–72
29. Lejeune F, Achten G (1983) Le mélanome malin cutané. Stratégies et résultats thérapeutiques. In: Le mélanome malin. XVIIe congrès de l'association des dermatologistes et syphiligraphes de langue française. Brussels, June 2–4, pp 249–291
30. Luck J (1956) Action of *p*-[di(2-chloroethylamino-L-phenylalanine] on Harding Passey mouse melanoma. Science 123:984–985
31. Martijn H, Olkhoff J, Schraffordt-Koops H, Oosterhuis J (1982) Hyperthermic regional perfusion with melphalan and a combination of melphalan and actinomycin D in the treatment of locally metastasized malignant melanoma of the extremities. J Surg Oncol 20:9–13
32. Martijn H, Oldhoff J, Oosterhuis JW, Schraffordt-Koops H (1983) Indications for elective groin dissection in clinical stage I patients with malignant melanoma of the lower extremity treated by hyperthermic regional perfusion. Cancer 52:1526–1534
33. Martijn H, Schraffordt-Koops H, Milton GW, Nap M, Oosterhuis JW, Shaw HM, Oldhoff J (1986) Comparison of two methods of treating primary malignant melanomas Clark IV et V, thickness 1.5 mm and greater localized on the extremities. Cancer 57:1923–1930
34. McBride CM, Sugarbaker EV, Hickey RC (1975) Prophylactic isolation perfusion as the primary therapy for invasive malignant melanoma of the limbs. Ann Surg 182:316–324
35. Millar RD, Ketcham AS (1974) The effect of heparin and warfarin on primary and metastatic tumors. J Med 5:23–31
36. Minor DR, Allen RE, Alberts D, Peng YM, Tardellin G, Hutchinson J (1985) A clinical and pharmacokinetic study of isolated limb perfusion with heat and melphalan for melanoma. Cancer 55:2638–2644
37. Nachbur B (1986) Die Perfusionsbehandlung des Extremitätenmelanomas. Indikationen, Technik, Komplikationen und Ergebnisse der regionalen Perfusionsbehandlung des malignen Melanomas der Extremitäten. Huber, Bern, p 104
38. Rampen FHJ (1985) Towards a rational perfusion strategy for malignant melanoma. Eur J Surg Oncol 11:117–118
39. Schraffordt-Koops H, Oldhoff J, Oosterhuis JW, Beekhuis H (1985) The role of isolated limb perfusion for regional metastases of the extremities. In: Balch CM (ed) Surgical approaches to cutaneous melanoma. Karger, Basel, pp 146–164 (Pigment Cell, vol 7.)
40. Shingleton WW, Seigler HF, Stocks LH, Downs RW (1975) Management of recurrent melanoma of the extremity. Cancer 35:574–579
41. Shiu MH, Knapper WH, Fortner JG, Yeh S, Horowitz G, Schnog J, Guerra J, Gould-Rossbach P, Ray C (1986) Regional isolated limb perfusion of melanoma in transit metastases using mechlorethamine (nitrogen mustard). J Clin Oncol 4:1819–1826
42. Stehlin JS (1969) Hyperthermic perfusion with chemotherapy for cancers of the extremity. Surg Gynecol Obstet 129:305–308
43. Stehlin JS, Giovanella BC, De Ipolyi PD, Muenz LR, Anderson RF (1975) Results of hyperthermic perfusion for melanoma of the extremities. Surg Gynecol Obstet 140:339–348
44. Storm FK, Morton DL (1985) Value of therapeutic hyperthermic limb perfusion in advanced recurrent melanoma of the lower extremity. Am J Surg 150:32–35
45. Storm FK, Silberman AW, Ramming KR, Kaiser LR, Harrison WH, Elliott RS, Haskell CM, Sarna G, Morton DL (1984) Clinical thermochemotherapy. A controlled trial in advanced cancer patients. Cancer 53:863–868
46. Sugarbaker ER, McBride CM (1976) Survival and regional disease control after isolation perfusion for invasive stage I melanoma of the extremities. Cancer 37:188–198
47. Sutherland CM, Mather FJ, Krementz ET (1987) Factors influencing the survival of patients with regional melanoma of the extremity treated by perfusion. Surg Gynecol Obstet 164:111–118
48. Tonak J, Hermanek P, Banz H, Groitl H (1979) Cytotoxics and hyperthermic perfusion: a preliminary study. Cancer Treat Rev 6:135–141
49. Tonak J, Hohenbergen W, Göhl J (1984) Die isolierte hypertherme Extremitätenperfusion bei malignen Melanomen und Weichgewebssarkomen. Chirurg 55:499–504
50. Van OS J, Schraffordt-Koops H, Oldhoff J (1985) Dosimetry of cytostatics in hyperthermic regional isolated perfusion. Cancer 55:698–701
51. Wagner DE (1976) A retrospective study of regional perfusion for melanoma. Arch Surg 111:410–413
52. Wieberding J, Benckhuysen C, Braat RP, Van Slooten EA, Olthuis GAA (1982) Dosimetry in isolation perfusion of the limbs by assessment of perfused tissue volume and grading of toxic tissue reactions. Eur J Cancer Clin Oncol 18:905–910

Subject Index

MIX
Papier aus verantwortungsvollen Quellen
Paper from responsible sources
FSC® C105338

If you have any concerns about our products,
you can contact us on
ProductSafety@springernature.com

In case Publisher is established outside the EU,
the EU authorized representative is:
Springer Nature Customer Service Center GmbH
Europaplatz 3, 69115 Heidelberg, Germany

Printed by Libri Plureos GmbH
in Hamburg, Germany